One Health and Zoonoses

One Health and Zoonoses

Special Issue Editors

John S. Mackenzie
Martyn Jeggo

MDPI • Basel • Beijing • Wuhan • Barcelona • Belgrade

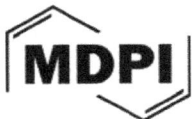

MDPI

Special Issue Editors

John S. Mackenzie
Curtin University Faculty of Health Sciences
Australia

Martyn Jeggo
AUSGEM Governing Board
Australia

Editorial Office
MDPI
St. Alban-Anlage 66
4052 Basel, Switzerland

This is a reprint of articles from the Special Issue published online in the open access journal *Tropical Medicine and Infectious Disease* (ISSN 2414-6366) in 2019 (available at: https://www.mdpi.com/journal/tropicalmed/special_issues/One_Health).

For citation purposes, cite each article independently as indicated on the article page online and as indicated below:

LastName, A.A.; LastName, B.B.; LastName, C.C. Article Title. *Journal Name* **Year**, *Article Number*, Page Range.

ISBN 978-3-03921-295-8 (Pbk)
ISBN 978-3-03921-296-5 (PDF)

Contents

About the Special Issue Editors

John S. Mackenzie, Professor, AO, FTSE, is an Emeritus Professor at Curtin University in Perth, Western Australia, where he held a Chair in Tropical Infectious Diseases. He is currently a part-time Senior Research Scientist at PathWest, Perth; an Honorary Professor in the School of Chemistry and Molecular Biosciences at the University of Queensland, St Lucia; and an Honorary Senior Principal Fellow at the Burnet Institute, Melbourne.

He has worked extensively with WHO, and particularly with the Global Outbreak Alert and Response Network, and the Asia Pacific Strategy for Emerging Infectious Diseases. He is a member of the Roster of Experts of the International Health Regulations. In 2009–2010, he was appointed as Chair of a WHO International Health Regulations Emergency Committee for Pandemic H1N1 influenza, and is currently a member of the International Health Regulations Emergency Committee Concerning the International Spread of Wild Poliovirus.

With his colleague, Prof. Martyn Jeggo, Mackenzie initiated the International One Health Congresses and helped to organize the first and fourth congresses in Melbourne. In 2015, he co-founded the One Health Platform Foundation with his colleagues Ab Osterhaus and Chris Vanlangendonck. The platform is a non-profit international foundation based in Belgium (www.onehealthplatform.com), and is responsible for the biennial World One Heath Congresses and the One Health Strategic Policy Forums.

Martyn Jeggo, Professor, BVetMed, FTSE, qualified as veterinary surgeon in the UK in 1972, and after a short four-year spell in general practice, has worked in research and the research management of infectious diseases. This included spells in a number of developing countries, at the UK high containment laboratory, and within the United Nations (UN). During this period of 18 years at the UN, he managed programs of support for animal health in the developing world, with research-related projects in some 150 countries. One such program involved support to laboratories in 40 countries and assisting in the global eradication of rinderpest. For this work, he was awarded a UN medal. In 2002, he became Director of the Australian Animal Health Laboratory and, as such, was a member of the Australian Animal Health Committee and Chair of SCHALS. In 2013, he retired from AAHL and now works on a part-time basis within the framework of the Geelong Centre for Emerging Infectious Diseases—a One Health consortium. He is Chair of the Governing Board of AUSGEM (a research partnership between UTS and EMAI, NSW), on the Board of the International Livestock Research Institute (ILRI), the Advisory Board of GALMED, and the International Advisory Board of SACIDS. For a number of years now, he has adopted a One Health approach to tackling a number of health research areas and along with Professor Mackenzie, has published a number of papers and books detailing the development and use of the One Health concept.

Preface to "One Health and Zoonoses"

The study of science began from the broadest possible base and was driven by the thinking man with little underlying specialized knowledge or formal education. As science understanding and science research developed, disciplines and areas of expertise developed, with specialized institutes, journals, funding, and even language. In the health arena, the broad disciplines of human medicine, veterinary medicine, and dentistry evolved, with the rapid development of many specialized areas of human medicine. This was fully warranted by the enormous amount of discipline-specific information, skills, qualifications, and outcomes that were required, enabling real progress to be made using targeted resources for specific problems to be resolved. But, over time, something was lost. The innovative understandings that can come from a comparative approach and the application of leanings from one discipline across to another became somewhat marginalized. The situation was made even worse, since a number of the big problems remaining—often called "wicked problems"—could only really be tackled through a multidisciplinary, multisectoral approach. This is precisely why a "One Health" approach has emerged in recent years, to tackle some of those health-related problems that have beguiled a focused disciplinary approach. The emergence of global avian influenza highlighted the value of a multisectoral, multidisciplinary approach, with the significant risks to humans being managed through effective interventions in poultry and in understanding of the role of wild birds as reservoir species. This required collaboration across very distinct sectors of agriculture, wildlife biology, and human health and, in many countries, paved the way for the adoption of a One Health approach across Government and in research, policy development, and field activities. A more focused example has been around the management of risks to Hendra, a bat-borne zoonotic virus that affects horses in Australia with a mortality rate of over 70%. In humans, it carries a similar lethal characteristic. Bringing together a One Health team of medical doctors, veterinarians, and ecologists, various options were considered. Killing all the bats in the vicinity was quickly dismissed, followed by the call for a human vaccine, given the time and cost involved. The concept of a vaccine to protect horses was developed, and resources focused on this outcome. Within 2 years, a commercial vaccine was in widespread use, resulting in both protection in horses and the removal of the risk to humans. Other complex problems in which a One Health approach is becoming a significant and effective mechanism are in antimicrobial resistance (AMR), and food safety and security. AMR is perhaps the most threatening problem facing the medical professions today. Possibly initiated but certainly exacerbated by misuse, both by the medical and veterinary professions, the problem exists across the world as a result of multiple causes, and requires a significant array of mitigating actions. The World Health Organization, the Food and Agriculture Organization, and the World Organization for Animal Health have collectively called for a One Health approach both to better understand the problem as well was to develop solutions that will work in a range of different settings. This indeed is a "wicked" problem requiring such an approach. This collection of papers serves to further demonstrate these approaches through highlighting research conducted on real world problems using a One Health approach.

John S. Mackenzie, Martyn Jeggo
Special Issue Editors

Tropical Medicine and
Infectious Disease

MDPI

Editorial

The One Health Approach—Why Is It So Important?

John S. Mackenzie [1,2,3,*] and **Martyn Jeggo** [4]

1   PathWest, Queen Elizabeth 2 Medical Centre, Nedlands, WA 6009, Australia
2   Faculty of Health Sciences, Curtin University, GPO Box U1987, Perth, WA 6845, Australia
3   One Health Platform Foundation, Overheet 48, 9290 Berlare, Belgium
4   AUSGEM Governing Board, 31 The Breakwater, Corlette, NSW 2315, Australia; jeggo.martyn@gmail.com
*   Correspondence: j.mackenzie@curtin.edu.au; Tel.: +61-439875697

Received: 28 May 2019; Accepted: 30 May 2019; Published: 31 May 2019

It has become increasingly clear over the past three decades that the majority of novel, emergent zoonotic infectious diseases originate in animals, especially wildlife [1], and that the principal drivers of their emergence are associated with human activities, including changes in ecosystems and land use, intensification of agriculture, urbanisation, and international travel and trade [2–6]. A collaborative and multi-disciplinary approach, cutting across boundaries of animal, human, and environmental health, is needed to understand the ecology of each emerging zoonotic disease in order to undertake a risk assessment, and to develop plans for response and control.

The term 'One Health' was first used in 2003–2004, and was associated with the emergence of severe acute respiratory disease (SARS) in early 2003 and subsequently by the spread of highly pathogenic avian influenza H5N1, and by the series of strategic goals known as the 'Manhattan Principles' derived at a meeting of the Wildlife Conservation Society in 2004, which clearly recognised the link between human and animal health and the threats that diseases pose to food supplies and economies. These principles were a vital step in recognising the critical importance of collaborative, cross-disciplinary approaches for responding to emerging and resurging diseases, and in particular, for the inclusion of wildlife health as an essential component of global disease prevention, surveillance, control, and mitigation [7].

The outbreak of SARS, the first severe and readily transmissible novel disease to emerge in the 21st century, led to the realisation that (a) a previously unknown pathogen could emerge from a wildlife source at any time and in any place and, without warning, threaten the health, well-being, and economies of all societies; (b) there was a clear need for countries to have the capability and capacity to maintain an effective alert and response system to detect and quickly react to outbreaks of international concern, and to share information about such outbreaks rapidly and transparently; and (c) responding to large multi-country outbreaks or pandemics requires global cooperation and global participation using the basic principles enshrined in One Health [8]. The emergence and spread of influenza H5N1 has been another excellent example of the importance of global cooperation and a One Health approach driven by the widespread concern that it might become the next influenza pandemic strain. It also served as a catalyst for the United Nations Secretary General to appoint a UN Systems Coordinator for Avian and Animal Influenza (UNSIC), and to form a major collaboration with a number of international and national organizations, including the World Health Organization (WHO), Food and Agriculture Organization (FAO), World Organization for Animal Health (OIE), United Nations Children's Fund (UNICEF), and World Bank and various national heath ministries, to develop the International Ministerial Conferences on Avian and Pandemic Influenza (IMCAPI). IMCAPI was a major driver in the surveillance and responses to influenza H5N1 [9] and subsequently in the development of a strategic framework built around a One Health approach that focussed on diminishing the risk and minimizing the global impact of epidemics and pandemics due to emerging infectious diseases [10].

The concept of One Health is not new and can be traced back for at least two hundred years [11], firstly as One Medicine, but then as One World, One Health and eventually One Health. There is no single, internationally agreed upon definition of One Health, although several have been suggested. The most commonly used definition shared by the US Centers for Disease Control and Prevention and the One Health Commission is: 'One Health is defined as a collaborative, multisectoral, and transdisciplinary approach—working at the local, regional, national, and global levels—with the goal of achieving optimal health outcomes recognizing the interconnection between people, animals, plants, and their shared environment'. A definition suggested by the One Health Global Network is: 'One Health recognizes that the health of humans, animals and ecosystems are interconnected. It involves applying a coordinated, collaborative, multidisciplinary and cross-sectoral approach to address potential or existing risks that originate at the animal-human-ecosystems interface'. A much simpler version of these two definitions is provided by the One Health Institute of the University of California at Davis: 'One Health is an approach to ensure the well-being of people, animals and the environment through collaborative problem solving—locally, nationally, and globally'. Others have a much broader view, as encapsulated in Figure 1.

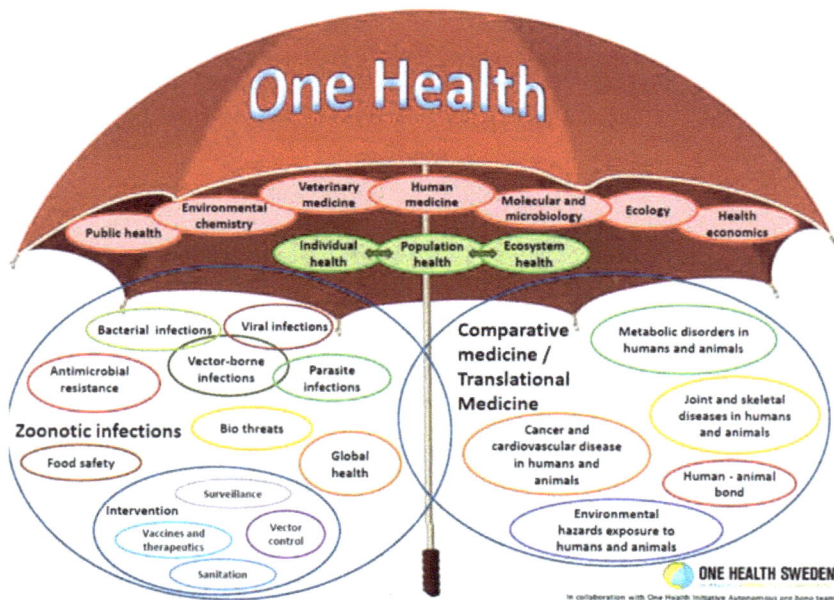

Figure 1. The One Health Umbrella, developed by One Health Sweden and the One Health Initiative Autonomous pro bono team.

The One Health concept clearly focusses on consequences, responses, and actions at the animal–human–ecosystems interfaces, and especially (a) emerging and endemic zoonoses, the latter being responsible for a much greater burden of disease in the developing world, with a major societal impact in resource-poor settings [12,13]; antimicrobial resistance (AMR), as resistance can arise in humans, animals, or the environment, and may spread from one to the other, and from one country to another [14–17]; and food safety [18,19]. However, the scope of One Health as envisaged by the international organizations (WHO, FAO, OIE, UNICEF), the World Bank, and many national organisations also clearly embraces other disciplines and domains, including environmental and ecosystem health, social sciences, ecology, wildlife, land use, and biodiversity. Interdisciplinary collaboration is at the heart of the One Health concept, but while the veterinarian community has embraced the One Health concept, the medical community has been much slower to fully engage, despite support for One Health from bodies such as the American Medical Association, Public Health England, and WHO. Engaging the medical community more fully in the future may require the incorporation of the One Health concept into the medical school curricula so that medical students see it as an essential component in the context of public health and infectious diseases [20].

One recent development that might help in generating increased global awareness of the One Health concept, particularly among students, but also more generally, has been the designation of November 3rd as One Health Day. Initiated in 2016 by the One Health Commission (www.onehealthcommission.org), the One Health Platform Foundation (www.onehealthplatform.com), and the One Health Initiative (http://www.onehealthinitiative.com), One Health Day is celebrated through One Health educational and awareness events held around the world. Students are especially encouraged to envision and implement One Health projects, and to enter them into an annual competition for the best student-led initiatives in each of four global regions.

Today's health problems are frequently complex, transboundary, multifactorial, and across species, and if approached from a purely medical, veterinary, or ecological standpoint, it is unlikely that sustainable mitigation strategies will be produced.

This special issue of *Tropical Medicine and Infectious Disease* contains a series of papers taking a One Health approach to a range of infectious diseases and the broader topic of antimicrobial resistance at the animal–human–environment interface, as well as to aspects of policy concerned with trade issues relating to AMR in the food chain and with aspects of public health policy and practice where significant knowledge gaps in the translation of scientific expertise and results, and biosafety and biosecurity measures, need to be addressed. These examples illustrate the critical importance of using a One Health approach for understanding and mitigating many current complex health problems. They demonstrate not only innovative approaches and outcomes but the range and types of collaborative partnerships that are required. This collection of papers demonstrates the breadth and scope of One Health, partly from an Australasian perspective, but also with an international flavour. They also serve to demonstrate the critical importance of taking a One Health approach to problems that have defied a more traditional disciplinary or sectoral approach.

Funding: This research received no external funding.

Conflicts of Interest: The authors declare no conflict of interest.

References

1. Taylor, L.H.; Latham, S.M.; Woolhouse, M.E. Risk factors for human disease emergence. *Philos. Trans. R. Soc. Lond. B Biol. Sci.* **2001**, *356*, 983–989. [CrossRef] [PubMed]
2. Lederberg, J.; Shope, R.E.; Oaks, S.C. (Eds.) *Institute of Medicine. Emerging Infections. Microbial Threats to the United States*; National Academy Press: Washington, DC, USA, 1992. Available online: https://www.ncbi.nlm.nih.gov/pubmed/25121245 (accessed on 23 May 2019).
3. Daszak, P.; Cunningham, A.A.; Hyatt, A.D. Anthropogenic environmental change and the emergence of infectious diseases in wildlife. *Acta Trop.* **2001**, *78*, 103–116. [CrossRef]
4. Jones, K.E.; Patel, N.G.; Levy, M.A.; Storeygard, A.; Balk, D.; Gittleman, J.L.; Daszak, P. Global trends in emerging infectious diseases. *Nature* **2008**, *451*, 990–993. [CrossRef] [PubMed]
5. Karesh, W.B.; Dobson, A.; Lloyd-Smith, J.O.; Lubroth, J.; Dixon, M.A.; Bennett, M.; Aldrich, S.; Harrington, T.; Formenty, P.; Loh, E.H.; et al. Ecology of zoonoses: Natural and unnatural histories. *Lancet* **2012**, *380*, 1936–1945. [CrossRef]
6. Jones, B.A.; Grace, D.; Kock, R.; Alonso, S.; Rushton, J.; Said, M.Y.; McKeever, D.; Mutua, F.; Young, J.; McDermott, J.; et al. Zoonosis emergence linked to agricultural intensification and environmental change. *Proc. Natl. Acad. Sci. USA* **2013**, *110*, 8399–8404. [CrossRef] [PubMed]
7. Wildlife Conservation Society. One World-One Health: Building Interdisciplinary Bridges. 2004. Available online: http://www.oneworldonehealth.org/sept2004/owoh_sept04.html (accessed on 22 May 2019).

8. Mackenzie, J.S.; McKinnon, M.; Jeggo, M. One Health: From Concept to Practice. In *Confronting Emerging Zoonoses: The One Health Paradigm*; Yamada, A., Kahn, L.H., Kaplan, B., Monath, T.P., Woodall, J., Conti, L., Eds.; Springer: Tokyo, Japan, 2014; pp. 163–189. [CrossRef]
9. IMCAPI. International Ministerial Conference: Animal and Pandemic Influenza: The Way Forward. In *Hanoi Declaration*; IMCAPI: Hanoi, Vietnam, 2010; Available online: http://www.un-influenza.org/?q=content/hanoi-declaration (accessed on 22 May 2019).
10. IMCAPI. Contributing to One World, One Health: A Strategic Framework for Risks of Infectious Diseases at the Animal-Human-Ecosystems Interface. Available online: http://www.fao.org/3/aj137e/aj137e00.pdf (accessed on 23 May 2019).
11. Atlas, R.M. One Health: Its origins and future. *Curr. Top. Microbiol. Immunol.* **2013**, *365*, 1–13. [CrossRef] [PubMed]
12. Cleaveland, S.; Sharp, J.; Abela-Ridder, B.; Allan, K.J.; Buza, J.; Crump, J.A.; Davis, A.; Del Rio Vilas, V.J.; de Glanville, W.A.; Kazwala, R.R.; et al. One Health contributions towards more effective and equitable approaches to health in low- and middle-income countries. *Philos. Trans. R. Soc. Lond. B Biol. Sci.* **2017**, *372*, 20160168. [CrossRef] [PubMed]
13. Welburn, S.C.; Beange, I.; Ducrotoy, M.J.; Okello, A.L. The neglected zoonoses–the case for integrated control and advocacy. *Clin. Microbiol. Infect.* **2015**, *21*, 433–443. [CrossRef] [PubMed]
14. WHO. WHO, FAO, and OIE Unite in the Fight Antimicrobial Resistance. Available online: https://www.who.int/foodsafety/areas_work/antimicrobial-resistance/amr_tripartite_flyer.pdf?ua=1 (accessed on 24 May 2019).
15. WHO. WHO Guidelines on Use of Medically Important Antimicrobials in Food-Producing Animals. Available online: https://apps.who.int/iris/bitstream/handle/10665/258970/9789241550130-eng.pdf;jsessionid=1853DF68D3CE5791633C651325955956?sequence=1 (accessed on 24 May 2019).
16. Hoelzer, K.; Wong, N.; Thomas, J.; Talkington, K.; Jungman, E.; Coukell, A. Antimicrobial drug use in food-producing animals and associated human health risks: What, and how strong, is the evidence? *BMC Vet. Res.* **2017**, *13*, 211. [CrossRef] [PubMed]
17. Ceric, O.; Tyson, G.H.; Goodman, L.B.; Mitchell, P.K.; Zhang, Y.; Prarat, M.; Cui, J.; Peak, L.; Scaria, J.; Antony, L.; et al. Enhancing the One Health initiative by using whole genome sequencing to monitor antimicrobial resistance of animal pathogens: Vet-LIRN collaborative project with veterinary diagnostic laboratories in United States and Canada. *BMC Vet. Res.* **2019**, *15*, 130. [CrossRef] [PubMed]
18. Garcia, S.N.; Osburn, B.I.; Cullor, J.S. A one health perspective on dairy production and dairy food safety. *One Health* **2019**, *7*, 100086. [CrossRef] [PubMed]
19. Boqvist, S.; Söderqvist, K.; Vågsholm, I. Food safety challenges and One Health. within Europe. *Acta Vet. Scand.* **2018**, *60*, 1. [CrossRef] [PubMed]
20. Rabinowitz, P.M.; Natterson-Horowitz, B.J.; Kahn, L.H.; Kock, R.; Pappaioanou, M. Incorporating one health into medical education. *BMC Med. Educ.* **2017**, *17*, 45. [CrossRef] [PubMed]

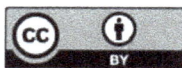

Tropical Medicine and Infectious Disease

MDPI

Article

Respiratory Illness in a Piggery Associated with the First Identified Outbreak of Swine Influenza in Australia: Assessing the Risk to Human Health and Zoonotic Potential

David W. Smith [1,2,*] , Ian G. Barr [3,4], Richmond Loh [5], Avram Levy [1], Simone Tempone [6], Mark O'Dea [7] , James Watson [8], Frank Y. K. Wong [8] and Paul V. Effler [2,6]

1. Department of Microbiology, PathWest Laboratory Medicine WA, Nedlands, WA 6009, Australia; avram.levy@health.wa.gov.au
2. Faculty of Health and Medical Sciences, University of Western Australia, Nedlands, WA 6009, Australia; paul.effler@health.wa.gov.au
3. World Health Organization (WHO) Collaborating Centre for Reference and Research on Influenza, at The Peter Doherty Institute for Infection and Immunity, Melbourne, VIC 3000, Australia; Ian.Barr@influenzacentre.org.au
4. Department of Microbiology and Immunology, University of Melbourne, at the Peter Doherty Institute for Infection and Immunity, Melbourne, VIC 3000, Australia
5. Sustainability and Biosecurity, Department of Primary Industries and Regional Development, Perth, WA 6151, Australia; richmond.loh@dpird.wa.gov.au
6. Communicable Disease Control Directorate, Department of Health Western Australia, Perth, WA 6004, Australia; simone.tempone@health.wa.gov.au
7. School of Veterinary Medicine, Murdoch University, Perth, WA 6150, Australia; M.ODea@murdoch.edu.au
8. CSIRO Australian Animal Health Laboratory, Geelong, VIC 3219, Australia; James.Watson@csiro.au (J.W.); Frank.Wong@csiro.au (F.Y.K.W.)
*   Correspondence: david.smith@health.wa.gov.au; Tel.: +61-863-834-438

Received: 17 May 2019; Accepted: 24 June 2019; Published: 25 June 2019

Abstract: Australia was previously believed to be free of enzootic swine influenza viruses due strict quarantine practices and use of biosecure breeding facilities. The first proven Australian outbreak of swine influenza occurred in Western Australian in 2012, revealing an unrecognized zoonotic risk, and a potential future pandemic threat. A public health investigation was undertaken to determine whether zoonotic infections had occurred and to reduce the risk of further transmission between humans and swine. A program of monitoring, testing, treatment, and vaccination was commenced, and a serosurvey of workers was also undertaken. No acute infections with the swine influenza viruses were detected. Serosurvey results were difficult to interpret due to previous influenza infections and past and current vaccinations. However, several workers had elevated haemagglutination inhibition (HI) antibody levels to the swine influenza viruses that could not be attributed to vaccination or infection with contemporaneous seasonal influenza A viruses. However, we lacked a suitable control population, so this was inconclusive. The experience was valuable in developing better protocols for managing outbreaks at the human–animal interface. Strict adherence to biosecurity practices, and ongoing monitoring of swine and their human contacts is important to mitigate pandemic risk. Strain specific serological assays would greatly assist in identifying zoonotic transmission.

Keywords: influenza; swine; Australia; human; pandemic

1. Introduction

Influenza A viruses (IAV) circulate and evolve continually within bird and swine populations of the world, and are known to be a source of sporadic zoonotic influenza infections, thus presenting a reservoir of potential human pandemic influenza strains. They are known to be present in domestic swine populations internationally, largely as a result of the virus being introduced from humans infected with seasonal influenza viruses [1–3]. Some of these human origin viruses persisted and evolved into stable swine lineages through genetic and antigenic drift and virus gene reassortment. They pose an ongoing potential threat to both animal and human health, as demonstrated by the 2009 pandemic, which arose from swine influenza viruses derived from both human and avian IAV that had undergone long term ongoing reassortment [4].

Human infections with swine IAV have been detected since the 1970s and have caused both sporadic cases and outbreaks, such as those reported in the USA [3,5,6]. These zoonotic viruses are mainly of the A(H3N2) subtype with some A(H1N1) and A(H1N2) viruses, which are referred to as variant viruses with a lower-case "v" placed after the subtype, e.g., A(H3N2)v to denote their swine origin.

Prior to 2012 it was believed that Australian domestic swine populations were free of swine lineages of IAV. This was ascribed to negative results from a few limited serosurveys, and the strict quarantine practices preventing importation of pigs and the use of biosecure breeding facilities for domestic swine within Australia. In 2009, a number of outbreaks due to A(H1N1)pdm09 occurred in domestic Australian swine populations through transmission from infected humans, and these have continued to occur sporadically ever since [7]. The virus had little or no apparent ill effect on the health of infected swine and there was no evidence that this resulted from, or led to, enzootic IAV in Australian swine, and so was not seen to be a threat to human or animal health nor a potential source of pandemic viruses.

However, in 2012 an outbreak of respiratory illness and death occurred amongst pigs in a biosecure piggery near Perth, the capital of Western Australia [8], shown to be due to several previously unidentified swine IAV containing genes of human origin [9]. A mild respiratory illness was also reported by several of the workers. A combined investigation of this outbreak by the Department of Agriculture and Food, Western Australia (DAFWA) and the Communicable Disease Control Directorate (CDCD) of the Department of Health Western Australia led to the detection of a number of genetically distinct divergent IAV in the swine.

An extensive phylogenetic analysis indicated that the IAV in the Western Australian swine contain human origin genes not found in human populations for several decades, and that they are distinct from those identified in swine in the rest of the world, including those subsequently identified in swine in a piggery in Queensland [9], approximately 4000 km distant. This ongoing circulation and evolution of IAV in the Western Australian swine population for up to several decades revealed an unrecognized potential zoonotic threat [9].

In view of the known risk of transmission of IAV from pigs to humans in other countries [2,6], interventions were undertaken to investigate and mitigate the risk of human infection. This paper describes the investigations undertaken into this outbreak to assess the potential risk to human contacts and to determine whether zoonotic transmission had occurred. The importance of these investigations has been further emphasized by the recent description of the first human infection with a variant swine H3N2, acquired within Australia [10]. This occurred outside Western Australia following exposure to exhibition swine at an agricultural fair, and was confirmed to be due to a virus similar to, but distinct from, the swine viruses found in Western Australian and Queensland swine.

2. Materials and Methods

Active surveillance for respiratory illness among the workers at the affected piggery was commenced when the outbreak was notified to the CDCD. Those who developed any respiratory illness were assessed by a medical practitioner, and mid-turbinate nasal and throat swabs were collected using flocked swabs (FLOQSwabs, Copan Diagnostic Inc, Murietta, CA, USA). Swab samples were placed in virus transport medium and transported to PathWest Laboratory Medicine WA (PathWest, Perth, Australia) at 4 °C. Serum samples from symptomatic individuals were collected by standard venipuncture, then stored and transported at 4 °C, with a convalescent sample collected 10–14 days later. Blood samples for the serosurvey were collected in the same manner.

PCR tests at PathWest used an in-house duplex assay which included specific real-time RT-PCRs, respectively, directed at the influenza A matrix gene, the seasonal A(H3N2) HA gene, the seasonal A(H1N1)pdm09 HA gene and the influenza B matrix gene [11]. PCR testing for other respiratory viruses in the human contacts was carried as previously described [12] and swabs were also inoculated onto an MDCK cell monolayer for virus isolation. Rhinovirus speciation was based on 5'NTR sequence [12] and the characterization of matrix, HA and NA genes of influenza A viruses was carried out by conventional Sanger sequencing.

Testing for antibodies to influenza A and B was performed by complement fixation titer (CFT) at PathWest, while haemagglutination inhibition (HI) antibody test for the human sera and the antigenic characterization of the swine IAV isolates was carried out at the World Health Organization Collaborating Centre for Reference and Research on Influenza (WHOCC), Melbourne, Victoria. Comparison of titers used a Kruskal–Wallis test performed on the $\log_2$ converted values.

3. Results

The outbreak of serious illness among swine began in mid-July 2012, and then gradually subsided over the course of a few weeks (Figure 1) [8].

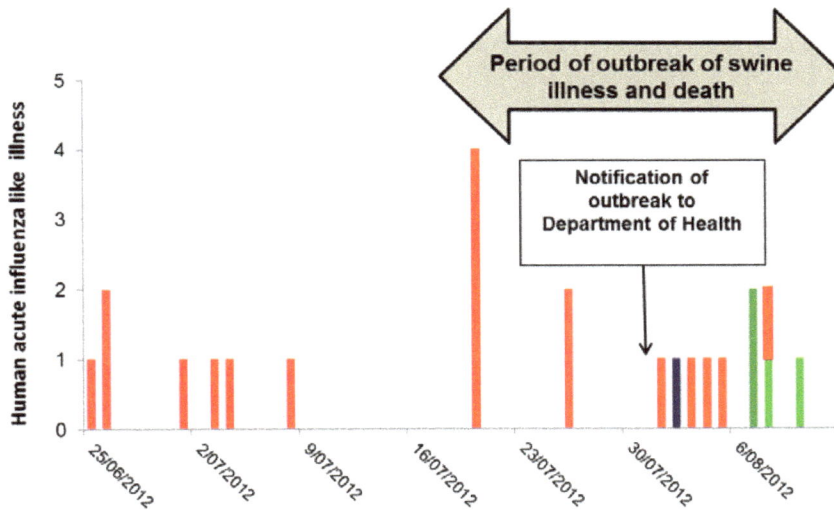

Figure 1. Date of onset of influenza-like illness and respiratory virus detections in 23 workers at a piggery in WA preceding and during an outbreak of respiratory tract illness and deaths in swine. The red columns are those with respiratory illness without laboratory confirmation either because they were not tested (17 workers) or because the results were negative or inconclusive. The blue column is confirmed seasonal A(H3N2) and the green are confirmed RV infections. Initial serologic testing at the DAFWA had suggested influenza infection and on 4 August 2012, a site visit was made by officers from the CDCD and the DAFWA.

No symptomatic humans were present during the initial site visit. However, 20 upper respiratory tract swabs were collected from symptomatic swine for testing by PCR and culture.

Initial PCR testing of the swine samples at PathWest were positive for influenza A matrix gene, but negative for the HA genes of the contemporaneously circulating A(H1N1)pdm09 and A(H3N2) viruses, indicating a possible novel HA type. This was later confirmed by the WHOCC in Melbourne and the Australian Animal Health Laboratories in Geelong, Victoria [9].

Following the initial testing, which indicated that these were likely to be nonseasonal IAV, suggesting a possible swine virus or an exotic human virus, the piggery was placed in quarantine [8] and surveillance for respiratory illness in staff at the piggery was commenced. A protocol was put in place to ensure that staff developing a respiratory illness were assessed and tested urgently by PCR, treatment with oral oseltamivir at 75mg twice daily was immediately provided, and the person was isolated at home until cleared of infection. Acute and convalescent serum samples were collected from these symptomatic workers and arrangements were made for collection of convalescent samples 10–14 days later. The use of personal protective equipment (PPE) by the staff in contact with swine was also emphasized, to reduce respiratory virus transmission.

Phylogenetic analysis of the swine IAVs characterized them as novel reassortant viruses containing only gene segments of human origin: two H1N2 reassortant viruses (H1N2/A/sw/WA/2577899R/2012 and H1N2/A/sw/WA/2577896X/2012) and one H3N2 reassortant virus (H3N2/A/Swine/WA/2577766G/2012) [9]. One of the A(H1N2) viruses (2577899R) and the A(H3N2) virus contained only segments that had not been detected in human populations for up to decades. These were chosen for the comparative serology. The other A(H1N2) virus (2577896X) had the same HA and NA genes as H1N2/2577899R, but the internal genes of the recent A(H1N1)pdm09 virus. The absence of any known matching viruses recently circulating in human populations internationally, and the ongoing circulation and evolution of these viruses within swine populations confirmed them as enzootic swine influenza viruses.

On 10 August, a week after the notification of the outbreak and following confirmation of the virus identification, seasonal influenza vaccination was carried out for the piggery workers, using the 2012 southern hemisphere trivalent influenza vaccine, and prophylaxis with oral oseltamivir 75 mg bd was provided for two weeks while vaccine responses were developing. This was done to reduce the risk of workers being infected with the variant virus, to reduce possible confounding seasonal influenza infections in the workers, to reduce the risk of further introduction of circulating human influenza viruses into the swine population, and to minimize the risk of mixed infections and reassortment between human and pig viruses [13].

Further testing of samples from 131 swine of various ages was carried out at PathWest in order to define the extent of the risk to human contacts. Of these, 43 (32.8%) had IAV detected based on a positive PCR for the matrix gene. Sanger sequencing of the products of the HA and NA genes indicated that six swine had a novel H1N2 virus, three (6.9%) had a novel H3N2 virus, one (2.3%) had A(H1N1)pdm09 infection, and two (4.6%) had likely seasonal A(H3N2) virus. The remainder could not be characterized by this sequencing. These results were consistent with whole genome sequencing result of the reassortant A(H1N2) and A(H3N2) swine viruses [9]. Sanger sequencing of the matrix gene of the six novel H1N2 viruses all matched with seasonal A(H1N1)pdm09 virus sequences, indicating that they were highly likely to be the H1N2/A/sw/WA/2577896X/2012 reassortant.

On 24 August 2012, three weeks after the notification of the outbreak to CDCD and two weeks after the vaccination program, 69 of 70 workers at the piggery completed a survey enquiring about symptoms of influenza-like illness during the period beginning one month prior to the outbreak in swine. Overall 27/69 (39%) of workers reported a mild respiratory illness in the month before or during the swine outbreak, and 23 of these 27 ill workers could recall their onset date. Seven had onset prior to the outbreak, seven during the swine outbreak but prior to notification, and nine after notification of the outbreak (Figure 1). Of those nine cases, eight were swabbed. One yielded a seasonal A(H3N2) virus, and three had a rhinovirus (RV), comprising two RV-C and one RV-A. The remaining four were negative for respiratory viruses.

Paired acute and convalescent serum samples were available for five cases (Table 1), including the individual with PCR-confirmed H3N2 infection who demonstrated an increase in HI antibodies to seasonal A(H3N2) from <1:10 to 1:320 between acute and convalescent sera, compared with an increase from 1:20 to 1:80 to the swine A(H3N2). Two others showed ≥ 4-fold rises in HI titers to A(H1N1)pdm09, one of whom also had a 4-fold rise in antibody titer to seasonal A(H3N2). However, both had been vaccinated between the acute and convalescent sample and this may have accounted for these results. The remaining workers did not show any significant HI changes.

Table 1. Acute and convalescent serum HI titers to swine and vaccine influenza A viruses for five workers with respiratory illness who provided acute and convalescent samples. Significant titer changes are in bolded text.

	Vaccine Given	Respiratory Illness between Samples	Sample	Swine Viruses		Vaccine Viruses	
				H1N2 A/WA/896X/2012	H3N2 A/WA/766G/2012	H1N1pdm09 A/California/7/2009	H3N2 A/Perth/16/2009
1	Yes	No	Acute	<10	10	<10	<10
			Convalescent	<10	<10	**320**	**40**
2	Yes	Yes [1]	Acute	<10	**20**	**10**	<10
			Convalescent	10	**80**	**40**	**320**
3	No	No	Acute	40	<10	20	20
			Convalescent	40	<10	40	10
4	Yes	No	Acute	20	20	40	80
			Convalescent	20	20	40	160
5	Yes	No	Acute	10	80	**40**	80
			Convalescent	**40**	160	**320**	160

[1] PCR-proven seasonal A(H3N2) infection.

Serum samples were requested at the time of the survey and 57/69 workers, 48 of whom had received the seasonal influenza vaccine two weeks earlier, agreed to provide serum samples. HI titers to swine A(H1N2) and A(H3N2) and to the vaccine A(H1N1) and A(H3N2) were determined (Table S1).

All of the nine unvaccinated workers had HI titers ≤1:80 to the swine A(H1N2) and all of these were lower than or equivalent to the titers to the vaccine A(H1N1). Seven had HI titers <40 to the swine A(H3N2), one had an HI titer of 40 to the swine A(H3N2) but this was lower than the titer to the vaccine A(H3N2). However, the remaining worker had a significantly higher HI titer to the swine A(H3N2) virus (1:320) than to the seasonal A(H3N2) virus (1:80). In summary, we found one unvaccinated worker who had serological evidence of a possible infection with the swine A(H3N2) virus. For the others, we either found no significant titers to the swine viruses or we could not exclude cross-reacting antibody due to infection with seasonal viruses, as represented by the vaccine strains.

The other 48 workers who underwent testing had received the seasonal influenza vaccine as part of the outbreak response. Therefore, we anticipated that we would detect vaccine-induced antibodies that might mask responses to infection with the swine viruses. Therefore we examined the likely effect of vaccination on antibody levels to the swine viruses by comparing HI titers in 48 vaccinated workers with those in the nine unvaccinated workers. Forty-six of the samples from vaccinated workers had sufficient volume to complete the testing for all viruses, while two further workers had sufficient sample to test for antibodies to the swine A(H1N2) and the vaccine A(H1N1) viruses, but not for antibodies to the A(H3N2) viruses (Table 2).

Vaccination had no effect on the HI titers to the swine A(H1N2) virus or the vaccine A(H1N1) strain, so that the antibody titers (Table S1) can be interpreted independent of vaccination. For the combined vaccinated and unvaccinated workers, there were a total of 24 workers who had HI titers ≥40 to the swine A(H1N2) virus, but 23 of these workers had equivalent or higher titers to the vaccine A(H1N1) virus, so that cross-reacting antibody from seasonal influenza A infection or vaccination could not be excluded. However, the remaining worker had a 16-fold higher titer to the swine A(H1N2) virus, suggesting possible infection with that virus.

In contrast, vaccination resulted in significant and similar increases in antibody titers to both the swine and seasonal A(H3N2) viruses. The results for the unvaccinated workers (see above) identified one worker with a possible swine A(H3N2) infection. Among the vaccinated workers, 35/46 had HI titers ≥40 to the swine A(H3N2) virus, of which 17 had higher titers to the swine virus than to the vaccine virus. Eight of these were only two-fold higher and were discounted as this difference was not significant. However, there were nine samples where the HI titer was between four-fold and 32-fold higher to the swine virus, which cannot be attributed to vaccination or seasonal virus infection.

Table 2. A comparison of the mean HI values in vaccinated and unvaccinated workers using a Kruskal–Wallis test on the $\log_2$-transformed HI titer, where HI titers <10 were assigned a notional value of 1. The one worker with a confirmed acute seasonal A(H3N2) infection was excluded.

Virus	Median of the $\log_2$-Converted HI Titers		*p*-Value
	Unvaccinated	Vaccinated [a]	
WA Swine H1N2 [1]	0.00	3.32	0.76
Human vaccine A/H1N1 09pdm [2]	6.32	6.32	0.87
WA Swine H3N2 [3]	3.32	6.32	0.0004
Human vaccine A/H3N2 [4]	5.32	6.32	0.025

[1] A/Swine/WA/2577896X/2012 H1N2, [2] A/California/7/2009 H1N1pdm09, [3] A/Swine/WA/2577766G/2012 H3N2, [4] A/Perth/16/2009 H3N2. [a] Only 46 workers were able to be tested for antibodies to the A(H3N2) viruses due to insufficient sample volume remaining for the final two workers.

These data suggest that, at least in some of the workers, there is evidence that they may have had an infection with one of the swine influenza viruses as their antibody titers could not be explained by cross-reacting antibody from their recent vaccination or seasonal influenza virus infection. However, we cannot exclude higher antibody titers due to past infection with human origin viruses that were serologically closely-related to the swine viruses, as we do not have a demographically matched control group that were not exposed to the swine influenza viruses.

4. Discussion

Influenza A viruses circulate and evolve continually within swine populations and represent a reservoir of potential human pandemic influenza strains. These viruses occasionally cross into human populations following contact with swine, including exhibition swine at agricultural events [6,14,15]. Until 2012 it was thought that Australia was free of this risk, as enzootic influenza had not been detected in local swine populations previously. Characterization of the outbreak described here clearly demonstrated that human influenza viruses have been regularly entering Australian swine populations from humans, probably for decades, and that circulation and reassortment has persisted within swine [9]. Infection of humans with variant influenza viruses arising from piggeries has not yet been documented, but there is a continuing possibility that swine viruses with pandemic potential may spread to humans in contact with swine within Australia. That appears to have happened with the recent first variant influenza virus infection of a human in Australia, associated with exposure to exhibition swine [10].

The Western Australian piggery outbreak was the first to identify enzootic influenza virus infection in swine in Australia [9], and we have described the approach taken to determine whether swine-to-human transmission had occurred and to mitigate the risk of further transmission between swine and humans. That included reinforcing personal hygiene measures and providing seasonal influenza vaccination for previously unvaccinated workers [16]. Active surveillance for respiratory illness in the workers was instituted as soon as the outbreak was notified, but none of the subsequent respiratory illnesses occurring could be attributed to the swine influenza viruses by PCR testing or by serology.

The limitations of using virus detection for assessing infection of human contacts are known, especially where long term exposure is likely and the illness is mild, so that the likelihood of identifying and sampling acute infections is low [17]. Serosurveys have the advantage of detecting past as well as current infections, but are problematic for influenza diagnosis due to the multiple exposures and vaccinations that occur during life and the cross-reactivity of influenza antibodies across different strains of the virus. Adults have diverse immune backgrounds to influenza and therefore have complex serological responses to infections with new influenza viruses. In our study, the interpretation of the results was further complicated by the vaccination program that had been undertaken two weeks prior to the serosurvey. This may have masked antibody responses to the swine viruses, which are difficult to separate from possible cross-reactions from the vaccine response and/or past natural exposure to human viruses.

However, we did not find any evidence that vaccination with the seasonal influenza vaccine influenced the antibody titer to the swine A(H1N2) virus. So the high titer HI antibody to this virus with a low titer to the seasonal A(H1N1)pdm09 virus that we found in one worker could not be explained by vaccination, and indicated possible infection with the swine virus. With the swine A(H3N2) viruses, we did find that vaccination increased titers to both the swine A(H3N2) and the vaccine A(H3N2) viruses, but several workers had HI titers to the swine A(H3N2) virus that were at least fourfold higher than the responses to the vaccine A(H3N2) virus. That result is not consistent with a vaccine response, and again suggests possible infection with a swine A(H3N2) virus. However, the HI titers to the swine A(H1N2) and A(H3N2) viruses could possibly have been due to past natural infection with antigenically similar viruses that circulated within human populations.

The challenges associated with using serosurveys to assess zoonotic influenza infections have been recently reviewed [17]. The authors recommended that, in order to identify antibodies specific to the animal viruses, the protocol should include testing for antibodies to both human and variant viruses for cross-reactivity; the use of two different serological assays, one of which should be a neutralization assay, to improve specificity; and having matched control samples from persons not in contact with the animals. Many of the piggery workers were from overseas, which meant that they had potentially been exposed to a different spectrum of influenza A viruses that may have resulted in antibodies that cross-reacted with the swine influenza viruses. Unfortunately, we could not access satisfactory control sera to exclude that possibility. In view of that limitation, we elected not to proceed with neutralization assays as it was unlikely to provide definitive results.

The ongoing circulation of influenza viruses within swine populations in Australia, with evidence of transmission between humans and swine overseas, and the likely recent human infection acquired within Australia has made us aware of potential for the generation of zoonotic infections. This also raises the possibility, albeit low, of human pandemic strains arising within Australia following zoonotic infection with a swine IAV. While commercial piggeries have not yet been shown to be a source of zoonotic infection with swine IAV, precautions are recommended to mitigate this risk [16]. Further studies are needed to identify the extent and diversity of influenza viruses in swine and other animals in regular contact with humans, and to conduct studies to determine the frequency of transmission to those human contacts.

The animal health sector has recently provided updated recommendations for maintaining biosecurity at piggeries, and for the management of outbreaks [18,19]. In addition it is important to restrict casual contact with swine at agricultural events, to carry out seasonal vaccination programs for piggery workers and others with regular swine contact, to maintain surveillance of people working at the human–animal interface and to have early structured investigation of outbreaks of respiratory illness in the animals or their human contacts [13,16].

Supplementary Materials: The following are available online at http://www.mdpi.com/2414-6366/4/2/96/s1, Table S1: HI values in vaccinated and unvaccinated workers. The one worker with a confirmed acute seasonal A(H1N2) infection was excluded. Highlighted results are those where the titer to a swine IAV was ≥40 and at least four-fold higher than the titer to the vaccine strain.

Trop. Med. Infect. Dis. **2019**, *4*, 96

Author Contributions: Conceptualization, D.W.S., P.V.E., and R.L.; Methodology, P.V.E., D.W.S., R.L., A.L., and M.O.; Formal Analysis, D.W.S., P.V.E., S.T., and I.J.B.; Investigation, P.V.E., R.L., S.T., and M.O.; Writing—Original Draft Preparation, D.W.S., P.V.E., and I.G.B.; Writing—Review & Editing, D.W.S., P.V.E., I.G.B., A.L., S.T., M.O., J.W. and F.Y.K.W.

Funding: This research received no external funding.

Acknowledgments: The authors would like to acknowledge the assistance and cooperation of staff at the Communicable Disease Control Directorate of the Health Department Western Australia, the Surveillance Unit at the Department of Microbiology, PathWest Laboratory Medicine WA at the QEII Medical Centre, the Department of Agriculture and Food Western Australia, and the World Health Organization Collaborating Centre for Reference and Research on Influenza, Melbourne.

Conflicts of Interest: The authors declare no conflicts of interest.

References

1. Myers, K.P.; Olsen, C.W.; Gray, G. Cases of swine influenza in humans: A review of the literature. *Clin. Infect. Dis.* **2007**, *44*, 1084–1088. [CrossRef] [PubMed]
2. Kitikoon, P.; Vincent, A.L.; Gauger, P.C.; Schlink, S.N.; Bayles, D.O.; Gramer, M.R.; Darnell, D.; Webby, R.; Lager, K.M.; Swenson, S.L.; et al. Pathogenicity and transmission in pigs of the novel A(H3N2)v influenza virus isolated from humans and characterization of swine H3N2 viruses isolated in 2010–2011. *J. Virol.* **2012**, *86*, 6804–6814. [CrossRef] [PubMed]
3. Baudon, E.; Peyre, M.; Peiris, M.; Cowling, B.J. Epidemiological features of influenza circulation in swine populations: A systematic review and meta-analysis. *PLoS ONE* **2017**, *12*, e0179044. [CrossRef] [PubMed]
4. Smith, G.J.; Vijaykrishna, D.; Bahl, J.; Lycett, S.J.; Worobey, M.; Pybus, O.G.; Ma, S.K.; Cheung, C.L.; Raghwani, J.; Bhatt, S.; et al. Origins and evolutionary genomics of the 2009 swine-origin H1N1 influenza A epidemic. *Nature* **2009**, *459*, 1122–1125. [CrossRef] [PubMed]
5. Vijaykrishna, D.; Smith, G.J.; Pybus, O.G.; Zhu, H.; Bhatt, S.; Poon, L.L.; Riley, S.; Bahl, J.; Ma, S.K.; Cheung, C.L.; et al. Long term evolution and transmission dynamics of swine influenza A virus. *Nature* **2011**, *473*, 519–522. [CrossRef] [PubMed]
6. Biggerstaff, M.; Reed, C.; Epperson, S.; Jhung, M.A.; Gambhir, M.; Bresee, J.S.; Jernigan, D.B.; Swerdlow, D.L.; Finelli, L. Estimates of the number of human infections with influenza A(H3N2) variant virus, United States, August 2011–April 2012. *Clin. Infect. Dis.* **2013**, *57* (Suppl. 1), S12–S15. [CrossRef] [PubMed]
7. Deng, Y.M.; Iannello, P.; Smith, I.; Watson, J.; Barr, I.G.; Daniels, P.; Komadina, N.; Harrower, B.; Wong, F.Y. Transmission of influenza A(H1N1) 2009 pandemic viruses in Australian swine. *Influenza Respir. Viruses* **2012**, *6*, e42-7. [CrossRef] [PubMed]
8. Webb, K. State and Territory Reports: Western Australia. *Anim. Health Surveill. Q. Rep.* **2012**, *17*, 19–20.
9. Wong, F.Y.K.; Donato, C.; Deng, Y.M.; Teng, D.; Komadina, N.; Baas, C.; Modak, J.; O'Dea, M.; Smith, D.W.; Effler, P.V.; et al. Divergent human-origin influenza viruses detected in Australian swine populations. *J. Virol.* **2018**, *92*, e00316-18. [CrossRef] [PubMed]
10. World Health Organization. Influenza at the human-animal interface: Summary and assessment, 22 January to 12 February 2019. 2019. Available online: www.who.int/influenza/human_animal_interface/Influenza_Summary_IRA_HA_interface_12_02_2019.pdf (accessed on 2 April 2019).
11. Chidlow, G.; Harnett, G.; Williams, S.; Levy, A.; Speers, D.; Smith, D.W. Duplex real-time RT-PCR assays for the rapid detection and identification of pandemic (H1N1) 2009 and seasonal influenza viruses A/H1, A/H3 and B. *J. Clin. Microbiol.* **2010**, *48*, 862–866. [CrossRef] [PubMed]
12. Chidlow, G.R.; Laing, I.A.; Harnett, G.B.; Greenhill, A.; Phuanukoonnon, S.; Siba, P.M.; Pomat, W.S.; Shellam, G.R.; Smith, D.W.; Lehmann, D. Respiratory viral pathogens associated with lower respiratory tract disease among young children in the highlands of Papua New Guinea. *J. Clin. Virol.* **2012**, *54*, 235–239. [CrossRef] [PubMed]
13. Centers for Disease Control. Interim Guidance for Workers Who Are Employed at Commercial Swine Farms: Preventing the Spread of Influenza a Viruses. Available online: https://www.cdc.gov/flu/swineflu/guidance-commercial-pigs.htm (accessed on 23 April 2019).
14. Baranovich, T.; Bahl, J. Influenza A virus diversity and transmission in exhibition swine. *J. Infect. Dis.* **2016**, *213*, 169–170. [CrossRef] [PubMed]

15. Wu, J.; Yi, L.; Ni, H.; Zou, L.; Zhang, H.; Zeng, X.; Liang, L.; Li, L.; Zhong, H.; Zhang, X.; et al. Anti-human H1N1pdm09 and swine H1N1 virus antibodies among swine workers in Guangdong Province, China. *Sci. Rep.* **2015**, *5*, 12507. [CrossRef] [PubMed]

16. Centers for Disease Control. Take Action to Prevent the Spread of flu Between Pigs and People. Available online: https://www.cdc.gov/flu/swineflu/prevention.htm (accessed on 3 April 2019).

17. Sikkema, R.; Freidl, G.; de Bruin, E.; Koopmans, M. Weighing serological evidence of human exposure to animal influenza viruses—a literature review. *Euro. Surveill.* **2016**, *21*, C30388. [CrossRef] [PubMed]

18. National Farm Biosecurity Manual for Pork Production. 2013. Available online: http://www.farmbiosecurity.com.au/wp-content/uploads/2013/08/National-Farm-Biosecurity-Manual-for-Pork-Production.pdf (accessed on 24 April 2019).

19. Animal Health Australia. AUSVETPLAN Response Policy Brief: Influenza A Viruses in Swine. Version 4.0 2018. Available online: //hdwa.health.wa.gov.au/users/home34/he08408/Downloads/FLU-SWINE-03-FINAL18May18-1.pdf (accessed on 24 April 2019).

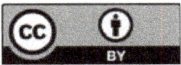

Tropical Medicine and Infectious Disease

MDPI

Article

Clinical and Epidemiological Patterns of Scrub Typhus, an Emerging Disease in Bhutan

Kezang Dorji [1,2]**, Yoenten Phuentshok** [1,3]🄳**, Tandin Zangpo** [1,4]**, Sithar Dorjee** [5]**,**
Chencho Dorjee [5]**, Peter Jolly** [1]**, Roger Morris** [6]**, Nelly Marquetoux** [1,*]🄳 **and Joanna McKenzie** [1]

[1]   School of Veterinary Science, Massey University, Palmerston North 4442, New Zealand;
        kezangt.dorjee@gmail.com (K.D.); vetyoen@gmail.com (Y.P.); zheynuapa@gmail.com (T.Z.);
        P.D.Jolly@massey.ac.nz (P.J.); J.S.McKenzie@massey.ac.nz (J.M.)
[2]   Samdrup Jongkhar Hospital, Ministry of Health, Samdrup Jongkhar 41001, Bhutan
[3]   National Centre for Animal Health, Department of Livestock, Ministry of Agriculture and Forests,
        Serbithang, Thimphu 11001, Bhutan
[4]   Dechencholing BHU-I, Ministry of Health, Thimphu 11001, Bhutan
[5]   Faculty of Nursing and Public Health, Khesar Gyalpo University of Medical Sciences of Bhutan,
        Thimphu 11001, Bhutan; s.dorjee@yahoo.co.nz (S.D.); director@rihs.edu.bt (C.D.)
[6]   Morvet Ltd., Consultancy Services in Health Risk Management and Food Safety Policy and Programs,
        Masterton 5885, New Zealand; roger.morris@morvet.co.nz
*   Correspondence: nelly.marquetoux@gmail.com; Tel.: +64-6-350-5701 (ext. 85755)

Received: 13 February 2019; Accepted: 18 March 2019; Published: 29 March 2019

Abstract: Scrub typhus (ST) is a vector-borne rickettsial infection causing acute febrile illness. The re-emergence of ST in the Asia-Pacific region represents a serious public health threat. ST was first detected in Bhutan in 2008. However, the disease is likely to be under-diagnosed and under-reported, and the true impact is difficult to estimate. At the end of 2014, the SD Bioline Tsutsugamushi Test™ rapid diagnostic test (RDT) kits became available in all hospitals to assist clinicians in diagnosing ST. We conducted a retrospective descriptive study, reviewing records from all hospitals of Bhutan to identify all RDT-positive clinical cases of ST in Bhutan in 2015. The aim was to evaluate the burden of ST in Bhutan, describe the demographic, spatial and temporal patterns of disease, and identify the typical clinical presentations. The annual incidence of RDT-positive cases of ST reporting to Bhutanese hospitals in 2015 was estimated to be 62 per 100,000 population at risk. The incidence of disease was highest in the southern districts with a subtropical climate and a high level of agricultural production. The highest proportion of cases (87%) was rural residents, with farmers being the main occupational category. The disease was strongly seasonal, with 97% of cases occurring between June and November, coinciding with the monsoon and agricultural production seasons. Common ST symptoms were not specific, and an eschar was noted by clinicians in only 7.4% of cases, which is likely to contribute to an under-diagnosis of ST. ST represents an important and neglected burden, especially in rural communities in Bhutan. The outcomes of this study will inform public health measures such as timely-awareness programmes for clinicians and the public in high-risk areas, to improve the diagnosis, treatment and clinical outcomes of this disease.

Keywords: scrub typhus; One Health; incidence; clinical pattern; descriptive epidemiology; vector-borne disease; emerging disease

1. Introduction

Scrub typhus (ST) or tsutsugamushi disease is a vector-borne rickettsial disease that is caused by the obligate intracellular bacterium *Orientia tsutsugamushi*. The primary reservoir is a trombiculid mite of the genus *Leptotrombidium*, which maintains the infection within populations through both transovarial and transtadial means of transmission [1]. Transmission to humans and other mammals occurs when the larval stage of infected mites feed on a human host [1]. A high risk of exposure to ST is associated with outdoor activities, agricultural work in particular, or living near grasslands or fields [2,3]. Humans are dead-end hosts, with no evidence of horizontal transmission of *O. tsutsugamushi* between people.

The geographic distribution of endemic ST is associated with the distribution of the reservoir mite in an area known as the 'tsutsugamushi triangle', centered on South-East and Pacific Asia [4]. ST has been described in this region for over a century [1,5]. The recent resurgence and re-emergence of ST in the endemic area has been associated with global climate change, influencing the distribution of infected mites [1]. Other putative factors are changes in agricultural practices and human behaviour, as well as improvements in diagnostic capabilities [5,6].

ST clinically presents as an acute non-specific febrile illness, which is difficult to diagnose [7]. Other common symptoms include nausea, vomiting, headache, myalgia and respiratory signs [8,9]. An eschar at the site of the bite, occurring before the onset of other symptoms, is pathognomonic [8,10]. However, the presence of an eschar, usually on the front of the body [11], is variably reported in 1–97% of ST patients, depending on the region of the world [1]. While ST is readily treated with antibiotics such as tetracycline, doxycycline, azithromycin and rifampicin [12], the nonspecific flu-like symptoms lead to the under-diagnosis and the under-treatment of this disease in many countries. Untreated ST can cause major complications and ultimately death. The median case fatality rate in untreated patients was estimated to be between 6 and 10% [1,13], but fatalities of up to 70% have been reported [1]. The duration of illness before effective antibiotic treatment is positively associated with progression to severe disease [14]. Hospital-based studies in South India reported a case fatality of 8–9% in ST patients reporting to the hospital, with multi-organ dysfunction observed in 34% of these patients [9,15]. Prompt clinical diagnosis and timely appropriate treatment are thus critical for improving the clinical outcome in individual patients [8,15], and for decreasing the public health impact of this disease [1].

In Bhutan, located within the tsutsugamushi triangle, ST was first identified as a cluster of pyrexia cases of unknown origin reporting to the Gedu hospital in the summer of 2008 [16]. A second outbreak occurred in Gedu in July 2009, of which 70% of cases were confirmed as ST by the Armed Forces Research Institute of Medical Sciences in Bangkok [17]. The disease was made notifiable in Bhutan in 2010. Notifications began to increase, particularly from the southern subtropical regions, which remain hot and humid for most of the year, and are exposed to the Indian summer monsoon [18]. However, given the non-specific presentation of ST, the disease was likely to be under-reported with only 22 to 67 cases being notified annually between 2012 and 2014. Misdiagnosis by clinicians and a lack of awareness amongst the public will respectively result in inappropriate case management, and delays in seeking treatment for febrile illness, in turn increasing the impact of ST in Bhutan.

In 2014, the Ministry of Health of Bhutan initiated a national sero-surveillance programme to gather more information on the incidence of ST, and to raise awareness among clinicians. In Bhutan, 19 of the 20 districts have a government district hospital, in which doctors provide in-patient and out-patient clinical services for the general public. The Gasa district in the far-north Himalayan area only has a Basic Healthcare Unit—Grade 1 (BHU-I) which functions as a district hospital. The country has two regional referral hospitals: in Gelephu, servicing southern Bhutan, and in Monggar, servicing eastern Bhutan. A national referral hospital is located in the capital city, Thimphu. There are no private medical services in Bhutan. As part of the sero-surveillance programme, the Ministry of Health approved the use of a commercial point-of-care rapid diagnostic test (RDT), the SD Bioline Tsutsugamushi Test™, in all hospitals and the BHU-I in Gasa, to support clinicians with the differential diagnosis and timely treatment of ST. The test has the advantage of low cost, rapidity, a single test result and simple interpretation [19]. The SD Bioline Tsutsugamushi Test™ is an immunochromatographic test that is designed for use in clinical settings. It detects IgM, IgG and IgA antibodies against *O. tsutsugamushi*, which increases the sensitivity of the test in patients that may seek treatment once past the acute phase, and those which have been re-infected with *O tsutsugamushi* and have an elevated IgG titre [20].

Under the national sero-surveillance programme, clinicians were encouraged to send samples from patients positive to the RDT to the Royal Centre for Disease Control (RCDC), which functions as the national public health laboratory in Thimphu, for confirmatory testing using the Scrub Typhus Detect TM IgM Enzyme-Linked Immunosorbent Assay (ELISA) test (Inbios International, Inc., Seattle, WA, USA). Cut-off values for the ELISA were calculated for samples collected from Bhutan with the assistance of a laboratory in Pune, India.

Before 2015, no population-wide information on ST was available in Bhutan. With new diagnostic capabilities becoming widely available in hospitals in 2015, a rise in diagnosed ST in Bhutan was expected, irrespective of the level of notification to the Ministry of Health. The aim of this descriptive epidemiology study was therefore to compile the first year of data that was generated by the improved diagnostic capability in hospitals and the national sero-surveillance programme, to gain insight into the epidemiological patterns of ST and the likely impact of ST in Bhutan.

The objectives of our study were to: (1) obtain a more accurate estimate of the incidence of clinical ST, (2) describe the clinical patterns of ST, and (3) describe the demographic, spatial and temporal epidemiological characteristics of clinical ST in Bhutan. The outcomes of this study would contribute to more accurate estimates of the national burden of disease, and support the development and implementation of public health measures to reduce the impact of ST.

2. Materials and Methods

We conducted a national descriptive study of laboratory-confirmed ST cases that were identified in hospitals in Bhutan in 2015. The case definition was clinically suspected ST cases that were confirmed by the Rapid Diagnostic Test (RDT; SD Bioline Tsutsugamushi Test^{TM}) during routine practice in hospitals in Bhutan during 2015.

2.1. Data Collection

ST cases were identified retrospectively by examining the clinical records of all district and referral hospitals and the BHU-I in Gasa district in early 2016. RDT-positive cases that were identified during a hospital-based case control study conducted from October to December 2015 in 11 districts with a higher incidence of ST were included. RDT-positive samples from this case-control study were sent to the RCDC for confirmatory IgM ELISA testing.

Data were obtained from RCDC on IgM ELISA-positive cases tested under the national sero-surveillance programme and the case control study.

For cases that were eligible for the case control study, demographic, clinical and epidemiological information were collected by interview during the study. For other patients, the clinical data were retrieved from the hospital records, and the demographic data was retrieved directly from the patient using their recorded contact details, where necessary.

The national census data issued by the Ministry of Health, Bhutan's Statistical Bureau, was used as the denominator to calculate national and district-level incidence, and age-based incidence rates of RDT-positive ST cases. The district population, as well as the rural versus urban population data was derived from 2015 statistics and age demographic data from 2017 statistics.

2.2. Analysis

We used descriptive methods to analyse the clinical and epidemiological characteristics of ST cases, including demographic, temporal and spatial distributions. Temporal patterns were based on the date of consultation in local hospitals. Spatial distribution was based on the address of the patient at the time of consultation. We mapped the district-level incidence of the RDT+ ST cases with and without the cases identified during the case control study, to identify a potential confounding of the case control study on the spatial distribution of ST. The age distribution between male and female patients was compared by using a two-sample Kolmogorov-Smirnov (KS) test. The proportion of patients experiencing each group of symptoms was compared between males and females using the Pearson's Chi-squared test. The proportion of rural versus urban cases was compared to that in the general population, using a test of equal proportions between samples.

Incidence rates were expressed as the cumulative number of ST cases per 100,000 persons at risk in 2015.

All analyses were performed using R [21].

2.3. Ethical Considerations

The ethical clearance was approved by the Research Ethics Board of Health (REBH), Ministry of Health, Royal Government of Bhutan, Thimphu via letter number REBH/PO/2015/042 on the 25 November 2015.

3. Results

A total of 470 RDT-positive clinical cases of ST was identified in this study, representing an observed annual incidence of 62 cases per 100,000 persons at risk in Bhutan in 2015. Among the 470 cases, 160 samples were sent to the RCDC for IgM ELISA testing, as part of the national sero-surveillance programme, of which 85 (53%) were ELISA-positive. A further subset of the 470 cases included 125 RDT-positive samples identified through the case control study which were tested with the IgM ELISA at RCDC, of which 79 (63%) were ELISA-positive.

There was a similar proportion of females (51.3%) and males (48.7%) among the cases. The median age of ST patients was 30 years old, with the highest percentage of cases within the 20–40-year-old period (Figure 1). The age distribution of ST in males and females was very similar (Figure 1) and statistically not different (KS p-value = 0.65). While the highest number of ST cases occurred in the 20–40-year old age group, the age-specific incidence was highest in age groups between 40 and 70 years old (Figure 2).

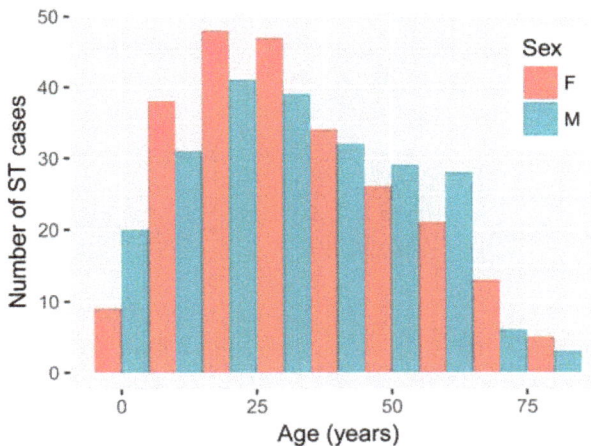

Figure 1. Age distribution of 470 clinically suspected scrub typhus (ST) cases that were positive to the SD Bioline Tsutsugamushi test in Bhutan in 2015.

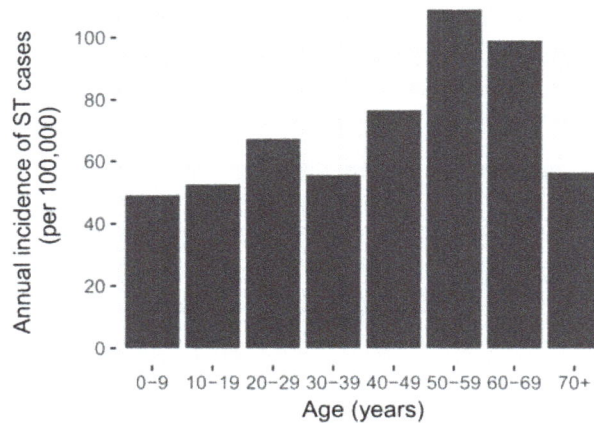

Figure 2. Age-specific incidences of 470 clinically suspected ST cases that were positive to the SD Bioline Tsutsugamushi test in Bhutan in 2015.

Farmers represented the main line of occupation among ST patients (45%), followed by students (22%) and housewives (17%) (Figure 3). The vast majority of patients were from rural areas (88%, *n* = 412) compared to 62% in the general population. Rural cases were overrepresented in the RDT-positive population, compared to the general population (*p* < 0.0001).

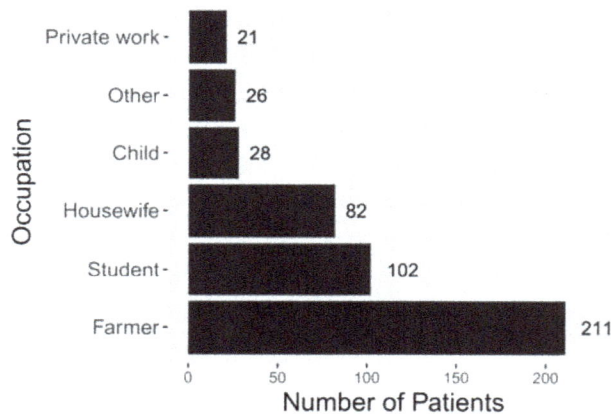

Figure 3. Occupation of 470 clinically suspected ST cases that were positive to the SD Bioline Tsutsugamushi test in Bhutan in 2015 (the "Other" category encompasses gomchen (lay priests), patients from India, military personnel, monks and civil servants).

The highest annual incidence of RDT-positive ST cases was observed in sub-tropical districts in the south of Bhutan (Figure 4). This spatial pattern was consistent with and without the cases identified through the case control study, which was conducted in the southern districts (Figure 4). Cases were observed in all districts except Gasa, which is located in the higher Himalayas.

a. Excluding 125 RDT–positive ST cases identified during the case–control study
conducted in 11 southern districts between October and December 2015

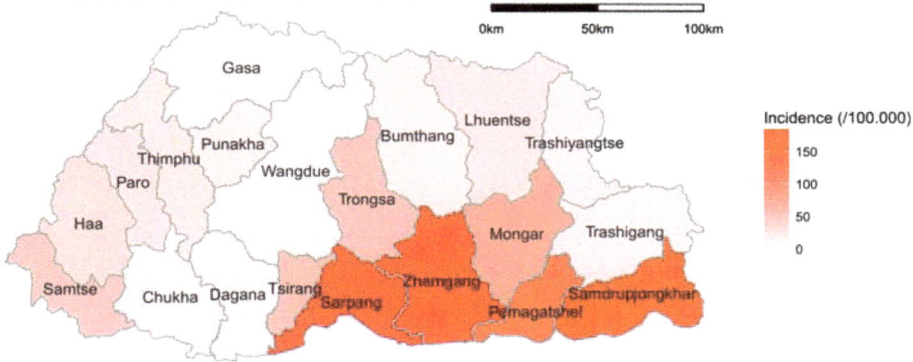

b. Including all 470 RDT–positive ST cases identified during 2015

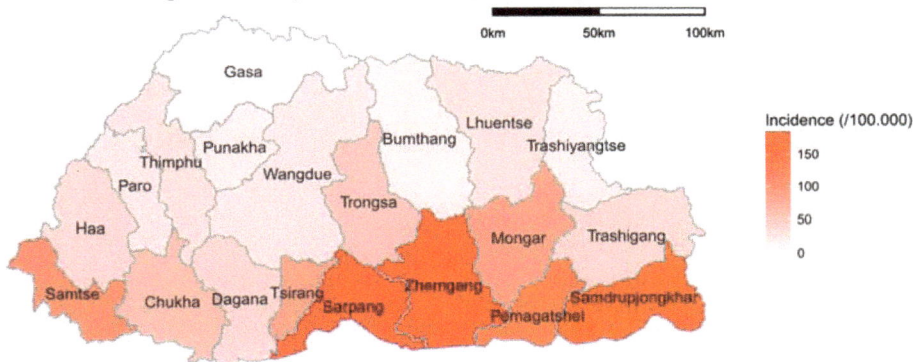

Figure 4. Spatial distribution of the incidences of clinically suspected scrub typhus cases that tested
positive to the SD Bioline Tsutsugamushi test in Bhutan in 2015 ((**a**) excluding 125 RDT-positive ST cases
that were identified during the case-control study conducted in 11 southern districts between October
and December 2015, (**b**) including all 470 RDT-positive ST cases that were identified during 2015).

The temporal distribution of ST cases showed a strong trend of seasonality that was associated
with the monsoon season. There were virtually no cases between December and June, followed by a
sharp increase in July with a peak of incidence in September, and a sudden drop from October onwards
(Figure 5).

Most RDT-positive ST cases presented with nonspecific flu-like symptoms. Fever was present
in all patients, since this was generally the criterion for clinicians to perform the RDT, headache in
87%, myalgia and poly-arthralgia, respectively, in 56% and 40% of patients, and diarrhea or vomiting
in 22% (Table 1). The presence of a pathognomonic eschar was only observed in 7.4% of the patients,
twice as commonly in males (10%) as females (5%) ($p = 0.06$). Males and females mostly presented
with a similar pattern of symptoms. However, respiratory and vascular symptoms were significantly
1.7 ($p = 0.01$) and 1.9 ($p = 0.04$) times more frequent in males.

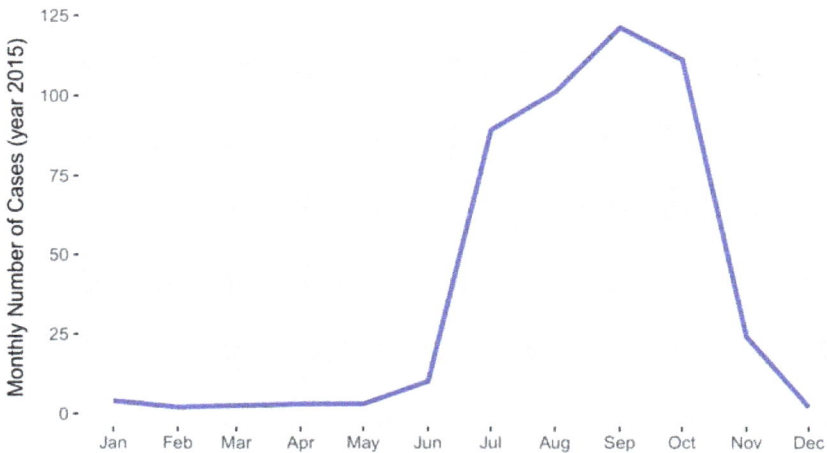

Figure 5. Temporal distribution of 470 clinically suspected scrub typhus cases that tested positive to the SD Bioline Tsutsugamushi test in Bhutan in 2015.

Table 1. Comparison of the clinical manifestations of 470 clinically suspected ST cases that tested positive to the SD Bioline Tsustugamushi test in males (241) and females (229) in Bhutan in 2015.

	Positive	*n*	Proportion (Overall)	Proportion (Males)	Proportion (Females)	*p*-Value
Fever	470	470	100%	100%	100%	NA
Headache	407	470	86.6%	83.8%	89.2%	0.12
Myalgia	265	470	56.4%	55.9%	56.8%	0.91
Malaise	216	468	46.2%	48.7%	43.8%	0.33
Polyarthralgia	189	470	40.2%	41.5%	39%	0.65
Other Digestive Symptoms	179	470	38.1%	37.1%	39%	0.74
Chills	130	469	27.7%	28.1%	27.4%	0.95
Diarrhoea/Vomiting	102	470	21.7%	21%	22.4%	0.79
Giddiness	95	467	20.3%	16.8%	23.7%	0.09
Respiratory Symptoms	91	470	19.4%	24.5%	14.5%	0.01
Rashes	88	469	18.8%	18.8%	18.8%	1
Vascular Symptoms	45	470	9.6%	12.7%	6.6%	0.04
Eschar	35	470	7.4%	10%	5%	0.06
Restlessness	31	470	6.6%	7%	6.2%	0.88
Lymphadenopathy	9	470	1.9%	2.2%	1.7%	0.94
Jaundice	3	470	0.6%	0.4%	0.8%	1

4. Discussion

The emergence of reported ST cases in Bhutan between 2010 and 2014 indicated the potential for ST to be a significant health issue in Bhutan. However, most healthcare workers as well as the public were not aware of the disease at that time. This is the first national study of ST in Bhutan, providing more accurate evidence for the overall incidence and the spatial, temporal and demographic distributions of ST in Bhutan's population in 2015.

The identification of 470 cases of RDT-positive ST in Bhutan in 2015, representing an observed annual incidence of 62 RDT-confirmed clinical ST cases/100,000 persons at risk, is a much higher incidence of ST than that reflected through the national sero-surveillance data from previous years. These results suggest that ST is a common cause of febrile illness in Bhutan. However, there are many challenges that are associated with serological testing for ST that make it difficult to interpret the extent to which this result reflects the true incidence of clinical ST in the Bhutanese population. Given the SD Bioline Tsutsugamushi test measures IgM, IgG and IgA antibodies it is likely to overestimate the incidence of clinical ST infections that occurred during 2015, given the test also captures antibodies that are associated with historical exposure in an unknown proportion of febrile cases [20]. This is supported by the IgM ELISA test results being positive in only 53% and 63% of the subset of RDT+ cases that were tested with the ELISA, respectively, in the sero-surveillance programme and the case control study. The IgM test results are likely to reflect the proportions of RDT+ cases that have current infections. The InBios Scrub Typhus Detect IgM ELISA was reported to have a sensitivity and specificity of 93% and 91% respectively, when measured against patients with typhus-like illness that fulfilled robust scrub typhus criteria in Thailand [22]. On the other hand, reinfection with *O. tsutsugamushi* is not uncommon in endemic areas, and such cases can be expected to have a rising IgG titre, which would not be captured in the IgM ELISA test results [20]. Furthermore, a proportion of cases who sought treatment after only a few days of fever may not have developed IgM antibodies, and this would have been missed by both serological tests [20]. In general, the RDT-positive incidence is more likely to reflect the overall exposure to *O. tsutsugamushi* amongst febrile patients, including recent and historical exposure, while the IgM ELISA incidence is more likely to reflect clinical disease that is associated with recent exposure. Both tests are likely to underestimate the true incidence of clinical ST in the study populations. Due to ST's non-specific flu-like symptoms, it is likely that not all cases would have sought treatment at the hospitals; milder or self-limiting cases of ST might not be seen in the hospital. The disease is also likely to be under-diagnosed, due to a lack of awareness of clinicians and non-specific clinical presentation. Moreover, anecdotal reports indicate that clinicians may have faced a shortage in the supply of RDT kits in some district hospitals in 2015, especially in high-incidence areas, and an unknown number of clinical ST cases may not have been tested.

There is considerable variation in the information on sensitivity and specificity of the SD Bioline Tsutsugamushi test. While the company selling the test claims a sensitivity and specificity of 99% and 96% respectively, one study evaluating this test against the immunofluorescence assay (IFA) in Thailand found a sensitivity of only 20.9% (95% CI: 10.0–36.0) in acute samples that are collected from patients who had a fever for a mean of 2–3 days. A higher sensitivity of 76.7% (95% CI: 61.4–88.2) was found in convalescent samples that were collected from the same patients at a median interval of 14 days (range 11–30 days). The specificity was similar in acute (74.4%; 95% CI: 58.8–86.5) and convalescent (76.7%; 95% CI: 61.4–88.2) samples [23]. Other studies have found that the same test had a sensitivity of 66.7% (95% CI 57.1–75.1%) and 72.6% in acute samples from febrile patients in Thailand and Korea, respectively, when assessed against the IFA [20,24]. Specificity was estimated to be 98.4% (95% CI: 91.5–99.7) in the Thai study [20]. Furthermore, there are acknowledged problems with evaluating the test accuracy by using the IFA as a gold standard, which may result in underestimates of sensitivity and specificity in the tests being evaluated [22]. The authors recommend the widespread use of the IgM ELISA, with optical density cut-offs, calibrated for an individual country, as a gold standard for the acute diagnosis of ST infections. The accuracy of serological tests may also be influenced by the variation in the circulating strains of *O. tsutsugamushi* [22,24]. The authors acknowledge the need for ST diagnostic tests to be validated within the country in which they are to be used, to provide more accurate results. The SD Bioline Tsutsugamushi test has not been validated for Bhutan, which further complicates the interpretation of how well the results represent the true ST situation in the country.

While there are challenges in interpreting how well the results of the RDT testing of clinically suspected ST cases reflect the true incidence of clinical ST in the national Bhutanese population, the results are reasonably comparable between sub-groups within the tested population, given that the same test was used throughout the country. It was previously thought that ST was endemic only in the southern part of the country. However, this study has shown that while the highest incidence of RDT-positive clinical ST cases occurred in the subtropical southern districts of Bhutan, cases occurred throughout Bhutan in all but one district, Gasa, which is located in the higher Himalaya area (Figure 4). Hence, ST is a vector-borne zoonotic disease of national importance. The higher incidence in subtropical areas is likely to be associated with the climate favouring the survival of chigger mites, together with higher levels of exposure to the vector through the more intensive farming activities undertaken in the favourable growing climate in this region. The lack of cases in the mountainous Gasa district may be due to an unsuitable environment for the reservoir's sustenance. However, it may also be influenced by the district not having a district-level hospital, which may have led to potential ST cases not being diagnosed and/or tested. Furthermore, the local population may experience difficulty in accessing medical services in this mountainous area, which could further contribute to an underestimation of the incidence of ST in this district.

There was a very strong temporal pattern in the occurrence of RDT-positive clinical ST cases, with 97% of cases observed between June and November, peaking in September (Figure 5). A similar pattern was found in a study in West Bengal, India [25]. This time of the year coincides with the monsoon and the cropping season, which might favour both the density of the chiggers and people's exposure to the vector through agricultural work.

The observed seasonal and spatial patterns of RDT-positive clinical ST cases could be affected by clinicians in high-risk areas having greater awareness of ST during the high-risk season. Data on the total number of clinically suspected ST cases and the number of cases tested with the RDT in hospitals were not available. Hence, we cannot assess the consistency with which the RDT was applied across the clinically suspected ST cases in all hospitals, nor the variation in the proportion of RDT-tested cases that were positive. However, it is unlikely that clinicians' prior knowledge of ST biased the results in this study. While clinicians in the southern areas of Bhutan are generally aware of a higher incidence of febrile disease during the monsoon season, they were mostly unaware of ST and its epidemiology at the time of the study, hence variable awareness of ST is unlikely to have had a significant effect on the clinical suspicion of ST, or the application of the RDT.

The case control study on clinical ST cases diagnosed from October to December 2015 in 11 districts in the south of Bhutan is likely to influence the observed spatial and temporal patterns, as clinicians would have had a greater awareness of ST during the study. Given the study did not begin until October 2015, it would not have influenced the increased incidence showing from July until the peak in September. Furthermore, it would provide more confidence that the incidence declined significantly in November and December. Mapping the RDT-positive ST cases without those from the case control study showed the same spatial pattern with a higher incidence in the southern districts of Bhutan. This gives confidence that there is a higher risk of ST in the subtropical southern districts of Bhutan. A possible source of bias in the spatial and temporal distribution of diagnosed ST may have arisen from a shortage of kits in some hospitals. There is no data available on the timing of diagnostic kit supply to district hospitals during 2015. However, anecdotal reports indicate that some hospitals experienced a temporary shortage of diagnostic kits, particularly hospitals in the high-incidence areas during the high-incidence time of year. This might have influenced the observed distribution of diagnosed cases.

ST predominantly affected people living in rural areas (87%), primarily farmers (45%) (Figure 3). This is consistent with previous observations throughout South-East Asia [25–28]. Students were the second-highest group with clinical ST. This is consistent with results from previous studies, highlighting the importance of ST in the differential diagnosis of children with pyrexia of unknown origin [29].

The highest age-specific incidence of clinical ST occurred in 40–70 year olds. The national statistics [30] show that a larger proportion of people aged 40 years and over live in rural areas (72%) compared with urban areas (28%). Hence, this age-related result is likely to be confounded with a higher risk of exposure of older people to rural environments and agricultural activities. It may also reflect the cumulative exposure of the at-risk population to *O. tsutsugamushi*, which is captured by the RDT measuring IgG and IgA, as well as IgM antibodies. Further studies that include multi-variable analyses would provide more accurate indications of the risk factors for ST.

Cases of ST in Bhutan presented as a nonspecific febrile illness, with signs of myalgia or poly-arthralgia in half the patients, consistent with reports in the literature [13,31]. Respiratory and vascular symptoms were significantly more frequent in males compared to females (respectively

1.7 and 1.9 times). Such a difference has not been reported in other studies, and it is difficult to propose an explanation for these differences. It may be confounded by variable distribution of these conditions between males and females in the over 40 year old age group. The presence of an eschar at the site of the chigger bite is described as pathognomonic [9], and it can thus be a precious diagnostic clue for clinicians. In Japan, 87% of patients presented with an eschar [27]. In contrast, this lesion was noted by the clinician in only 7.4% of patients (10% in males and 5% in females) in the present study. It is possible that clinicians did not thoroughly investigate patients for this lesion, especially female patients. The low detection rate of eschars may also be influenced by the inclusion of febrile patients with historical exposure to ST in the RDT-positive population, given the test measures of IgG and IgA, as well as IgM antibodies.

Among the 470 RDT-positive cases identified in hospitals, samples from only 160 cases were submitted from only four hospitals to the RCDC under the national sero-surveillance programme. The hospitals were: the national referral hospital in Thimphu, the regional referral hospitals in Sarpang and Mongar, and the secondary referral hospital in Paro. District hospitals in the rest of the country did not contribute samples, due to the perceived difficulty of transporting the samples to Thimphu, and a general lack of awareness about the sero-surveillance programme. As a result, the data generated through the national sero-surveillance programme significantly under-represents the true incidence of clinical ST in Bhutan. Raising clinicians' awareness of the sero-surveillance programme and ensuring facilities are available to transport samples from district hospitals to the RCDC in Thimphu would improve the representativeness of the sero-surveillance data. This would improve the ability of the Ministry of Health to monitor trends and to determine if clinical ST continues to emerge over time and over geographic areas in Bhutan. It would also indicate hospitals that may be under-diagnosing ST, which would enable targeted measures to be implemented to improve treatment-seeking behaviours of the public, and/or the diagnosis and treatment of ST in such areas where there is a difference between the expected and actual reported cases.

Despite the limitations of the SD Bioline Tsutsugamushi test, such commercial point of care tests are considered to be useful in clinical settings in limited resource environments to guide the differential diagnosis of ST [32], with the advantages of affordability, rapidity, single test results and ease of interpretation [19]. However, the tests need to be used with appropriate clinical discernment. It is important for clinicians to rule out other causes of acute febrile illness and the possibility of co-infection of patients with other infections that are associated with similar exposures, such as dengue and other rickettsial diseases. Given the limitations in the sensitivity of the test, clinicians should be encouraged to initiate treatment in patients in which they strongly suspect ST, even if the sample tests negative to the RDT, and to send samples from such patients to RCDC for confirmatory testing with the IgM ELISA. The epidemiological information generated through this study provides supplementary information that clinicians can use to diagnose ST, even in the absence of a positive RDT. Furthermore, epidemiological information can significantly contribute to the formulation and timely implementation of public health measures to reduce the burden of ST in Bhutan. Communication programmes can be implemented in all areas, to raise the awareness of the public to seek treatment if they are suffering flu-like symptoms. Likewise, providing clinicians with guidelines and professional training in risk factors for ST, such as the times of year, geographic areas, occupations and types of exposure to potential chigger habitat could increase the probability of considering ST in the differential diagnosis for patients presenting with nonspecific febrile illness. The timely supply of test kits and therapeutic drugs to hospitals, especially in high-risk areas, may contribute to the improved diagnosis and treatment of ST cases.

This study represents an important step towards understanding the incidence and associated risk factors for ST in Bhutan, which can inform both public health measures and the design of future studies. It would be valuable to validate the SD Bioline Tsutsugamushi test in Bhutan. Furthermore, studies to identify the antigenic variants of *O. tsutsugamushi* in Bhutan and in neighbouring areas of northern India could help with the development of more sensitive serological tests. Given the complex nature of this vector-borne zoonotic disease, One Health studies, involving collaboration between multiple sectors and disciplines, are required to explore the roles of the environmental and anthropologic factors, and the ecology of the reservoir and vector population, to understand the drivers of the spatial, temporal and demographic distributions of ST in Bhutan.

Author Contributions: Conceptualisation, K.D., Y.P., T.Z., S.D., N.M. and J.M.; Data curation, K.D., Y.P., T.Z. and N.M.; Formal analysis, N.M.; Funding acquisition, P.J. and R.M.; Investigation, K.D., Y.P. and T.Z.; Methodology, K.D., S.D., N.M. and J.M.; Project administration, K.D., S.D., C.D. and J.M.; Resources, C.D., P.J., R.M. and J.M.; Supervision, S.D., P.J., R.M. and J.M.; Validation, K.D., Y.P., T.Z. and N.M.; Visualization, N.M.; Writing—original draft, K.D., Y.P., T.Z. and S.D.; Writing—review & editing, P.J., N.M. and J.M.

Funding: This study received funding from the European Union through the One Health program in Asia (europeaid/133708/c/act/multi; contract dci-asie/2013/331-217).

Acknowledgments: We acknowledge the dedicated support of the district health staff who were instrumental in this study. The program was implemented by Massey University, in collaboration with Khesar Gyalpo University of Medical Sciences, and the Royal University of Bhutan.

Conflicts of Interest: The authors declare there are no conflicts of interest.

References

1. Xu, G.; Walker, D.H.; Jupiter, D.; Melby, P.C.; Arcari, C.M. A review of the global epidemiology of scrub typhus. *PLoS Negl. Trop. Dis.* **2017**, *11*, e0006062. [CrossRef] [PubMed]
2. Lyu, Y.; Tian, L.; Zhang, L.; Dou, X.; Wang, X.; Li, W.; Zhang, X.; Sun, Y.; Guan, Z.; Li, X.; et al. A Case-Control Study of Risk Factors Associated with Scrub Typhus Infection in Beijing, China. *PLoS ONE* **2013**, *8*, e63668. [CrossRef]
3. Newton, P.N.; Day, N.P. 63—Scrub Typhus. In *Hunter's Tropical Medicine and Emerging Infectious Disease*, 9th ed.; Magill, A.J., Hill, D.R., Solomon, T., Ryan, E.T., Eds.; W.B. Saunders: London, UK, 2013; pp. 542–545.
4. Yang, H.-H.; Huang, I.-T.; Lin, C.-H.; Chen, T.-Y.; Chen, L.-K. New Genotypes of *Orientia tsutsugamushi* Isolated from Humans in Eastern Taiwan. *PLoS ONE* **2012**, *7*, e46997. [CrossRef] [PubMed]
5. Chakraborty, S.; Sarma, N. Scrub Typhus: An Emerging Threat. *Indian J. Dermatol.* **2017**, *62*, 478–485. [PubMed]
6. Wei, Y.; Huang, Y.; Li, X.; Ma, Y.; Tao, X.; Wu, X.; Yang, Z. Climate variability, animal reservoir and transmission of scrub typhus in Southern China. *PLoS Negl. Trop. Dis.* **2017**, *11*, e0005447. [CrossRef]
7. Chang, K.; Lee, N.-Y.; Ko, W.-C.; Tsai, J.-J.; Lin, W.-R.; Chen, T.-C.; Lu, P.-L.; Chen, Y.-H. Identification of factors for physicians to facilitate early differential diagnosis of scrub typhus, murine typhus, and Q fever from dengue fever in Taiwan. *J. Microbiol. Immunol. Infect.* **2017**, *50*, 104–111. [CrossRef]
8. Rajapakse, S.; Rodrigo, C.; Fernando, D. Scrub typhus: Pathophysiology, clinical manifestations and prognosis. *Asian Pac. J. Trop. Med.* **2012**, *5*, 261–264. [CrossRef]
9. Varghese, G.M.; Trowbridge, P.; Janardhanan, J.; Thomas, K.; Peter, J.V.; Mathews, P.; Abraham, O.C.; Kavitha, M. Clinical profile and improving mortality trend of scrub typhus in South India. *Int. J. Infect. Dis.* **2014**, *23*, 39–43. [CrossRef]
10. Jeong, Y.J.; Kim, S.; Wook, Y.D.; Lee, J.W.; Kim, K.-I.; Lee, S.H. Scrub Typhus: Clinical, Pathologic, and Imaging Findings1. *Radio Graph.* **2007**, *27*, 161–172. [CrossRef]
11. Kim, D.-M.; Shin, H.; Lee, S.-H.; Song, H.-J.; Park, C.Y.; Lee, J.H.; Kim, H.S.; Kim, H.K.; Won, K.J.; Yang, T.Y.; et al. Distribution of eschars on the body of scrub typhus patients: A prospective study. *Am. J. Trop. Med. Hyg.* **2007**, *76*, 806–809. [CrossRef]
12. El Sayed, I.; Liu, Q.; Wee, I.; Hine, P. Antibiotics for treating scrub typhus. *Cochrane Database Syst. Rev.* **2018**. [CrossRef] [PubMed]
13. Paris, D.H.; Shelite, T.R.; Day, N.P.; Walker, D.H. Unresolved Problems Related to Scrub Typhus: A Seriously Neglected Life-Threatening Disease. *Am. J. Trop. Med. Hyg.* **2013**, *89*, 301–307. [CrossRef]
14. Zhang, L.; Zhao, Z.; Bi, Z.; Kou, Z.; Zhang, M.; Yang, L.; Zheng, L. Risk factors associated with severe scrub typhus in Shandong, northern China. *Int. J. Infect. Dis.* **2014**, *29*, 203–207. [CrossRef]

15. Varghese, G.M.; Janardhanan, J.; Trowbridge, P.; Peter, J.V.; Prakash, J.A.; Sathyendra, S.; Thomas, K.; David, T.S.; Kavitha, M.; Abraham, O.C.; et al. Scrub typhus in South India: Clinical and laboratory manifestations, genetic variability, and outcome. *Int. J. Infectious Dis.* **2013**, *17*, e981–e987. [CrossRef] [PubMed]

16. Dorji, T.; Wangchuk, S.; Lhazeen, K. Clinical Characteristics of Scrub Typhus in Gedu and Mongar (Bhutan). 2010. Available online: http://www.rcdc.gov.bt/web/clinical-characteristics-of-scrub-typhus-in-gedu-and-mongarbhutan/ (accessed on 4 April 2018).

17. Tshokey, T.; Choden, T.; Sharma, R. Scrub typhus in Bhutan: A synthesis of data from 2009 to 2014. *WHO South East Asia J. Public Health* **2016**, *5*, 117. [CrossRef]

18. Banerjee, A.; Bandopadhyay, R. Biodiversity Hotspot of Bhutan and its Sustainability. *Curr. Sci.* **2016**, *110*, 521. [CrossRef]

19. Shivalli, S. Diagnostic evaluation of rapid tests for scrub typhus in the Indian population is needed. *Infect. Dis. Poverty* **2016**, *5*, 894. [CrossRef] [PubMed]

20. Silpasakorn, S.; Waywa, D.; Hoontrakul, S.; Suttinont, C.; Losuwanaluk, K.; Suputtamongkol, Y. Performance of SD Bioline Tsutsugamushi assays for the diagnosis of scrub typhus in Thailand. *J. Med. Assoc. Thai* **2012**, *95*, 5.

21. R Development Core Team. *R: A Language and Environment for Statistical Computing*; R Foundation for Statistical Computing: Vienna, Austria, 2014.

22. Blacksell, S.D.; Tanganuchitcharnchai, A.; Nawtaisong, P.; Kantipong, P.; Laongnualpanich, A.; Day, N.P.J.; Paris, D.H. Diagnostic Accuracy of the InBios Scrub Typhus Detect Enzyme-Linked Immunoassay for the Detection of IgM Antibodies in Northern Thailand. *Clin. Vaccine Immunol.* **2016**, *23*, 148–154. [CrossRef] [PubMed]

23. Watthanaworawit, W.; Hanboonkunupakarn, B.; Nosten, F.; Tanganuchitcharnchai, A.; Jintaworn, S.; Blacksell, S.D.; Turner, P.; Turner, C.; Richards, A.L.; Day, N.P.J. Diagnostic Accuracy Assessment of Immunochromatographic Tests for the Rapid Detection of Antibodies against *Orientia tsutsugamushi* Using Paired Acute and Convalescent Specimens. *Am. J. Trop. Med. Hyg.* **2015**, *93*, 1168–1171. [CrossRef]

24. Lee, K.-D.; Moon, C.; Oh, W.S.; Sohn, K.M.; Kim, B.-N. Diagnosis of scrub typhus: Introduction of the immunochromatographic test in Korea. *Korean J. Intern. Med.* **2014**, *29*, 253–255. [CrossRef] [PubMed]

25. Sharma, P.K.; Ramakrishnan, R.; Hutin, Y.; Barui, A.; Manickam, P.; Kakkar, M.; Mittal, V.; Gupte, M. Scrub typhus in Darjeeling, India: Opportunities for simple, practical prevention measures. *Trans. R. Soc. Trop. Med. Hyg.* **2009**, *103*, 1153–1158. [CrossRef]

26. Lee, Y.-S.; Wang, P.-H.; Tseng, S.-J.; Ko, C.-F.; Teng, H.-J. Epidemiology of scrub typhus in eastern Taiwan, 2000–2004. *Jpn. J. Infect. Dis.* **2006**, *59*, 235–238. [PubMed]

27. Ogawa, M.; Hagiwara, T.; Kishimoto, T.; Shiga, S.; Yoshida, Y.; Furuya, Y.; Kaiho, I.; Ito, T.; Nemoto, H.; Yamamoto, N.; et al. Scrub typhus in Japan: Epidemiology and clinical features of cases reported in 1998. *Am. J. Trop. Med. Hyg.* **2002**, *67*, 162–165. [CrossRef]

28. Vallée, J.; Thaojaikong, T.; Moore, C.E.; Phetsouvanh, R.; Richards, A.L.; Souris, M.; Fournet, F.; Salem, G.; Gonzalez, J.-P.J.; Newton, P.N. Contrasting Spatial Distribution and Risk Factors for Past Infection with Scrub Typhus and Murine Typhus in Vientiane City, Lao PDR. *PLOS Negl. Trop. Dis.* **2010**, *4*, e909. [CrossRef]

29. Yadav, D.; Chopra, A.; Dutta, A.K.; Kumar, S.; Kumar, V. Scrub Typhus: An Uncommon Cause of Pyrexia without Focus. *J. Nepal Paedtr. Soc.* **2013**, *33*, 234–235. [CrossRef]

30. National Statistics Bureau. *Population Projections for Bhutan 2017–2047*; Royal Government of Bhutan: Thimphu, Bhutan, 2019.

31. Rapsang, A.G.; Bhattacharyya, P. Scrub typhus. *Indian J. Anaesth.* **2013**, *57*, 127. [PubMed]

32. Chanana, L.; Atre, K.; Galwankar, S.; Kelkar, D. State of the Globe: What's the Right Test for Diagnosing Rickettseal Diseases. *J. Glob. Infect. Dis.* **2016**, *8*, 95–96. [CrossRef] [PubMed]

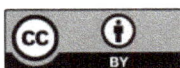

Tropical Medicine and Infectious Disease

MDPI

Article

Risk Factors for *Brucella* Seroprevalence in Peri-Urban Dairy Farms in Five Indian Cities

Johanna F. Lindahl [1,2,3], Jatinder Paul Singh Gill [4], Razibuddin Ahmed Hazarika [5], Nadeem Mohamed Fairoze [6], Jasbir S. Bedi [4], Ian Dohoo [7], Abhimanyu Singh Chauhan [8,9], Delia Grace [1] and Manish Kakkar [8,*]

[1]   Department of Biosciences, International Livestock Research Institute, Nairobi 00100, Kenya;
      J.lindahl@cgiar.org (J.F.L.); D.Randolph@cgiar.org (D.G.)
[2]   Department of Clinical Sciences, Swedish University of Agricultural Sciences, PO Box 7054,
      SE-750 07 Uppsala, Sweden
[3]   Zoonosis Science Centre, Department of Medical Biochemistry and Microbiology, Uppsala University,
      Po Box 582, SE-751 23 Uppsala, Sweden
[4]   Guru Angad Dev Veterinary and Animal Sciences University, Ludhiana 141004, Punjab, India;
      gilljps@gmail.com (J.P.S.G.); bedijasbir78@gmail.com (J.S.B.)
[5]   Department of Veterinary Public Health, Assam Agricultural University, Khanapara Campus,
      Guwahati-781022, India; rah1962@rediffmail.com
[6]   Department of LPT, Veterinary College, Karnataka Veterinary Animal & Fisheries Sciences University
      Bangalore, Bangalore 560024, India; prof.nadeem@gmail.com
[7]   Atlantic Veterinary College, University of Prince Edward Island, Charlottetown, C1A 4P3, Canada;
      dohoo@upei.ca
[8]   Public Health Foundation India, Gurgaon 122002, India; abhimanyu.hm@gmail.com
[9]   Department of Public Health Sciences, Faculty of Medicine, University of Liège, 4000 Liege, Belgium
*   Correspondence: manish.kakkar@phfi.org; Tel.: +91-124-4781400

Received: 15 March 2019; Accepted: 17 April 2019; Published: 22 April 2019

Abstract: Brucellosis is endemic among dairy animals in India, contributing to production losses and posing a health risk to people, especially farmers and others in close contact with dairy animals or their products. Growing urban populations demand increased milk supplies, resulting in intensifying dairy production at the peri-urban fringe. Peri-urban dairying is under-studied but has implications for disease transmission, both positive and negative. In this cross-sectional study, five Indian cities were selected to represent different geographies and urbanization extent. Around each, we randomly selected 34 peri-urban villages, and in each village three smallholder dairy farms (defined as having a maximum of 10 dairy animals) were randomly selected. The farmers were interviewed, and milk samples were taken from up to three animals. These were tested using a commercial ELISA for antibodies against *Brucella abortus*, and factors associated with herd seroprevalence were identified. In all, 164 out of 1163 cows (14.1%, 95% CI 12.2–16.2%) were seropositive for *Brucella*. In total, 91 out of 510 farms (17.8%, 95% CI 14.6–21.4%) had at least one positive animal, and out of these, just seven farmers stated that they had vaccinated against brucellosis. In four cities, the farm-level seroprevalence ranged between 1.4–5.2%, while the fifth city had a seroprevalence of 72.5%. This city had larger, zero-grazing herds, used artificial insemination to a much higher degree, replaced their animals by purchasing from their neighbors, were less likely to contact a veterinarian in case of sick animals, and were also judged to be less clean. Within the high-prevalence city, farms were at higher risk of being infected if they had a young owner and if they were judged less clean. In the low-prevalence cities, no risk factors could be identified. In conclusion, this study has identified that a city can have a high burden of infected animals in the peri-urban areas, but that seroprevalence is strongly influenced by the husbandry system. Increased intensification can be associated with increased risk, and thus the practices associated with this, such as artificial insemination, are also associated with increased risk. These results may be important to identify high-risk areas for prioritizing interventions and for policy decisions influencing the structure and development of the dairy industry.

Keywords: zoonoses; prevalence; *Brucella abortus*; urban livestock keeping; smallholder farming

---

1. Introduction

Infectious diseases cause a major burden on both human health and society as a whole. Zoonotic diseases inflict a double burden, since they also affect animal health, with associated costs and reduced productivity. Brucellosis is a very common but frequently neglected zoonosis that occurs globally, except for in a few countries that have managed to eradicate it, and the disease is often underreported and uncontrolled in low and middle-income countries, which may have the highest burden of the disease [1–4].

The disease can be caused by different bacteria of the genus *Brucella*, of which most species are pathogenic to multiple mammals, including cattle and humans [5,6]. Cattle are most frequently infected by *Brucella abortus* or *Brucella melitensis* [5,6]. These bacteria cause a chronic infection with preferred localization in the reproductive system, where they can cause abortion in pregnant cows or other reproductive problems, as well as reduced milk production in lactating animals and orchitis in bulls [1,7]. Although most infected animals only abort once, they may remain infected their entire life [8]. After the first abortion, as well as in non-pregnant animals, the disease can be asymptomatic [5]. Infected male cattle can spread the disease sexually, and both sexes may become infertile. Joint hygromas are another common manifestation of brucellosis [3].

Milk consumption has been increasing in low and middle-income countries, a trend likely to continue as the demand for animal-source food trends upwards due to population growth, changing lifestyles, and increasing wealth [9]. In India, the large vegetarian population increases the dependence on dairy products for high quality proteins. India has the world's largest dairy herd at around 300 million and is the world's leading milk producer, contributing around 17% of the world's total milk production, with more than 70 million households engaged in milk production [10,11]. Milk consumption is higher in urban areas and while the majority of the Indian population still live in rural areas, urbanization is increasing. Cities require a constant supply of fresh milk, and peri-urban dairy production plays an important role in meeting this demand.

The health of livestock, humans and livelihoods are closely linked, with zoonotic diseases such as brucellosis causing not only human and animal morbidity, but also reduced animal production and hence reduced incomes [12,13]. In India, awareness of brucellosis is low among livestock-keepers and healthcare staff, and because of the non-specific symptoms and the limited availability of laboratory facilities in many rural hospitals, diagnosis is seldom feasible [14,15]. Multiple studies have found seropositivity in humans in India, indicating the need to have an OneHealth approach for controlling this disease [16].

2. Materials and Methods

2.1. Ethical Approval

The study received ethical approval from the ethics committee of the Public Health Foundation of India [TRC-IEC-219/14, 27 May 2014; amended 12 October 2015]. Ethical approval was also obtained by Institutional Ethics Committees of Guru Angad Dev Veterinary and Animal Sciences University (GADVASU), Assam Agricultural University (AAU), Karnataka Veterinary, Animal and Fisheries Sciences University (KVAFSU), Rajasthan University of Veterinary and Animal Sciences (RAJUVAS) and School of Biotechnology, Kalinga Institute of Industrial Technology (KSBT) at the Ludhiana, Guwahati, Bangalore, Udaipur and Bhubaneswar study sites, respectively. Before a farmer was interviewed, they were informed about the purpose of the study and gave their consent to participate.

2.2. Farm Selection

Five Indian cities were selected purposively to represent different parts of the country (Figure 1). Peri-urban was defined as within 5 km of the official city boundaries, and all villages in that circle were mapped. For the purpose of this study, smallholder farms were defined as a dairy farm with a herd size of less than 10 cattle/buffaloes at the time of the survey and at least one milking animal, with dairy constituting a source of livelihood with or without domestic consumption. A systematic selection of 34 of these villages was done by identifying the proportion that needed to be sampled, and then systematically choosing these in a clockwise fashion around the city. The selected villages were then visited to identify all farms, using local village leaders as guides. The methodology of the creation of this sampling frame has been described elsewhere [17]. Out of this sampling frame, three smallholder farmers per village were randomly selected.

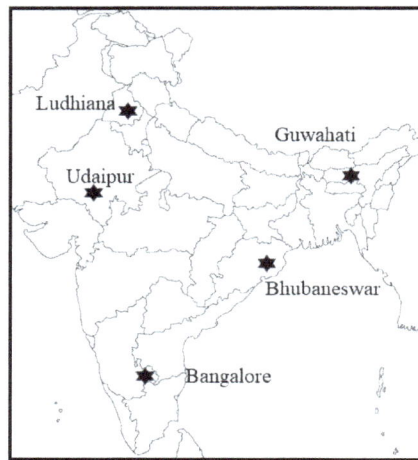

Figure 1. Location of selected cities in India.

2.3. Data Collection

Data collection was done between June 2015 and January 2016. A questionnaire was developed and piloted on farms in each site before starting the sampling. The tool was uploaded into electronic format and data collection was conducted using tablets, from which the data was uploaded into a central server. Data was collected by different data collection teams in each city, but all teams were trained by the same trainers, who joined in the first days of data collection. The data was collected through interviews in the local language, after the participants had been read the information about the project and given their written consent. Observations about cleaning practices and hygienic status were done during milking using an observation checklist. Cleanliness and drainage scores were standardized using pictures to guide the grading, and the scoring was assessed during the training to make sure it was consistent. Knowledge about antibiotics was assessed based on if the farmer reported to know the word (in the local language).

2.4. Sample Collection

In each farm, up to three milking cows or buffaloes were selected for sampling. In the 33% of farms where the number of milking cattle exceeded three, all cows were given a unique number, and then three numbers were selected randomly. The data collection teams were trained on aseptic collection of milk from the selected cows, and 40 mL of milk was collected in sterile vials and immediately kept chilled until they were transported to the laboratory on the same day of collection. The samples were thereafter stored in deep freezer at −80 °C. Samples were kept frozen when transported to the laboratory of microbiology at GADVASU and stored at −80 °C until analysis.

2.5. Serological Analysis

Milk was analyzed for the presence of antibodies using a commercial indirect enzyme-linked immunosorbent assay (iELISA) developed for use with milk samples (IDEXX Brucellosis Milk X2 Ab Test, IDEXX, Westbrook, ME, USA). The protocol of the manufacturer was followed, and all samples were done in duplicates. In brief, 50 µL of milk was diluted into 200 µL of sample diluent on a microplate precoated with *Brucella* lipopolysaccharide (LPS). The plate was incubated for 90 min, before being washed and the subsequent addition of conjugated anti-bovine IgG antibodies. After 30 min of incubation and washing, the tetramethylbenzidine (TMB) substrate was added and incubated for 20 min before the stop solution was added and the plate read at 450 nm.

The ratio of the optical density of the samples (mean) to the mean positive control was calculated after subtracting the mean of the negative controls from both. A ratio of above 55% was considered positive, while between 45 and 55% was considered suspected positive. In the analysis, only one sample was suspected positive, and since all other animals tested at the same farm were also positive, this animal is considered positive in the analyses and results. The specificity for this kit used on milk samples has been found to be very high [18], and a meta-analysis suggest a specificity of 96% for ELISA conducted on milk [19].

2.6. Data Analysis

An initial screening of all information collected was carried out with only the variables listed in Table 1 being retained for analysis, after identifying the variables with potential causal association with brucellosis. Analysis of the retained data proceeded in four steps. First, multiple correspondence analysis (MCA) was used to investigate relationships among all the predictors recorded. All predictors were initially recoded to di- or trichotomous variables. An MCA was carried out using all predictors and those having a contribution to either the first or second dimension that exceeded 0.02 were retained. The process was repeated sequentially with the required contribution being raised by 0.01 at each step (to a maximum of 0.06). At this point, the six variables that best explained the information content of the full set had been identified and these were plotted on a two-dimensional MCA plot (Figure 2).

One site (Guwahati) had a dramatically higher farm prevalence (72%) than the other four sites (4%), so the second step in the analysis was to evaluate the unconditional associations between each of the predictors and a variable representing Guwahati compared to the other sites. Either two-sample *t*-tests or cross-tabulations with chi-square statistics were used to determine if the regions were different. Results are presented in Table 1. Guwahati was also added as a supplemental variable (s51 vs s50 in Figure 2) to the MCA plot in Figure 2 to show which predictors were most associated with Guwahati vs other sites.

The third step was to use logistic regression models to identify factors associated with the risk of a farm being *Brucella* spp. positive within Guwahati, using backward elimination among variables with unconditional associations with $p < 0.15$. A random effect for village was included in all models. The linearity of continuous predictors was evaluated using lowess smoothed curves and a quadratic term was added to the model if there was significant evidence of curvature in the relationship. Initially, unconditional associations were determined with predictors having $p < 0.15$ retained for further consideration. A manual backward elimination was used to remove non-significant (at $p > 0.05$) predictors. Age of farmer and farm size (number of animals) were forced into all models as potential confounders. In addition to age and number of animals, two factors (cleanliness of floor and level of vaccination) were identified as potentially important. An MCA plot was generated (using trichotomous versions of each of the predictors) with *Brucella* spp. added as a supplemental variable to the final plot to see which predictors were generally associated with being *Brucella* spp. positive or negative.

Table 1. Potential risk factors for brucellosis given as either mean (standard deviation), or proportion (95% confidence interval).

	All Sites	Guwahati	Bangalore	Bhubaneswar	Ludhiana	Udaipur	p-Value *
Age of farmer	46.2 (12.3)	43.9 (12.9)	44.8 (13.2)	51.1 (10.8)	46.6 (12.7)	44.6 (10.2)	0.035
Female respondents	21.8% (18.3–25.6)	15.7% (9.2–24.2)	41.2% (31.5–51.4)	11.8% (6.2–19.6)	14.7% (8.5–23.1)	25.5% (17.4–35.1)	0.096
Illiterate respondents	35.4% (31.0–39.9)	51.1% (40.2–61.9)	41.1% (30.8–52.0)	23.5% (15.7–33.0)	15.7% (8.6–25.3)	44.9% (34.8–55.3)	0.001
Number of dairy animals	7.7 (4.0)	10.3 (4.1)	5.4 (2.7)	8.1 (3.6)	7.2 (3.7)	7.5 (4.0)	<0.001
Zero-grazing	53.3% (48.9–57.7)	95.1% (88.9–98.3)	9.8% (4.8–17.2)	4.9% (1.6–11.1)	93.1% (86.4–97.2)	63.7% (53.6–73.0)	<0.001
Using AI	76.0% (72.1–79.7)	92.2% (85.1–96.6)	98.0% (93.1–99.8%)	47.5% (37.5–57.7)	69.6% (59.7–78.3)	72.5% (62.8–80.9)	<0.001
Purchasing cows from neighboring farms	57.6% (52.8–62.3)	98.9% (94.0–100)	71.7% (57.7–83.2)	21.1% (13.4–30.6)	34.4% (24.9–45.0)	69.0% (59.0–77.9)	<0.001
Dirty floors in cow sheds	11.1% (8.5–14.2)	24.8% (16.7–34.3)	11.0% (5.6–18.8)	10.8% (5.5–18.5)	6.1% (2.3–12.7)	3.0% (0.6–8.4)	<0.001
Well-drained floors	19.8% (16.4–23.6)	8.9% (4.2–16.2)	22.8% (15.2–32.5)	23.5% (15.7–33.0)	35.4% (26.0–45.6)	8.9% (4.2–16.2)	0.007
Never vaccinate animals	15.5% (12.4–18.9)	25.5% (17.4–35.1)	0% (0–3.6)	2.0% (0.2–6.9)	7.8% (3.4–14.9)	42.42% (32.4–52.3)	<0.001
Vaccinate young animals routinely	26.7% (22.9–30.7)	61.8% (51.6–71.2)	2.9% (0.6–8.4)	44.1% (34.3–54.3)	0% (0–3.6)	24.5% (16.5–34.0)	<0.001
Records of sick animals	11.6% (8.0–14.7)	0% (0–3.6)	8.8% (4.1–16.1)	24.5% (16.5–34.0)	1.0% (0–5.3)	23.5% (15.7–33.0)	<0.001
Alpha score for cleaning routines	2.19 (0.28)	2.14 (0.23)	2.10 (0.28)	2.16 (0.08)	2.06 (0.13)	2.50 (0.34)	0.034
Alpha score for observed hygiene	0.32 (0.28)	0.10 (0.11)	0.31 (0.21)	0.60 (0.31)	0.25 (0.21)	0.35 (0.23)	<0.001
Regular health checks	23.9% (20.3–27.9)	3.9% (1.1–9.7)	14.7% (8.5–23.1)	33.3% (24.3–43.4)	46.1% (36.2–56.2)	21.6% (14.0–30.8)	<0.001
Let veterinarian check animals before purchase, or test the animal	25.9% (22.1–29.9)	2.9% (0.6–8.4)	35.3% (26.1–45.4)	58.8% (48.6–68.5)	9.8% (4.8–17.3)	22.6% (14.9–31.9)	<0.001
Quarantine new animals	24.6% (20.8–28.4)	17.7% (10.8–26.4)	19.6% (12.4–28.6)	41.4% (31.6–51.8)	19.6% (12.4–28.6)	24.5% (16.5–34.0)	0.074

* Comparing Guwahati with the four other sites.

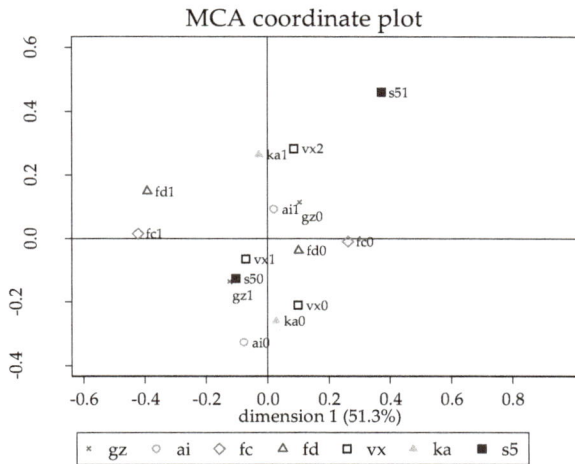

Figure 2. Multiple correspondence analysis (MCA) plot for the factors associated with the high seroprevalence site. Gz = grazing, where gz0 is zero-grazing and gz1 is grazing. Ai = artificial insemination, where ai0 is no artificial insemination and ai1 is use of artificial insemination. Fc = floor cleanliness, where fc0 is clean or moderately clean floor and fc1 is dirty floor. Fd = drainage, where fd0 equals insufficient drainage and fd1 is good drainage. Vx = vaccination, where vx0 means no vaccination done, vx1 means vaccination when there is an outbreak or when given free vaccines, and vx2 means vaccinating animals as young. Ka = knowledge about antibiotics, where ka0 is no knowledge and ka1 is the farmer reporting to know about antibiotics. S5 = site Guwahati, where s50 means any other site and s51 means Guwahati.

Finally, the model building process was repeated to determine which factors most influenced the risk of being *Brucella* spp. positive in sites 1 to 4. Only two predictors (farm size and use of *Haemorrhagic septicemia* vaccine) had unconditional associations with $p < 0.15$, but neither of these was significant in a final model so no results are presented.

3. Results

3.1. Brucella Seroprevalence

In total, 164 out of 1163 cows (14.1%, 95% CI 12.2–16.2%) were seropositive for *Brucella*.

A farm was considered positive for *Brucella* if at least one out of the three tested animals tested positive. In total, 91 farms out of 510 (17.8%, 95% CI 14.6%–21.4%) had at least one positive animal (see Table 2), and out of these, 23 farms had two positive animals and 25 (all in Guwahati) had all three animals positive. There were large differences in farm prevalence between the five different cities (Table 2). Guwahati had significantly higher seroprevalence ($p < 0.001$) than the other sites, and the odds ratio for a farm being positive in Guwahati was 44.4 (95% CI 7.5–113.2) times higher than in Udaipur and 138.9 (95% CI 32.0–602.3) times higher than in Bhubaneswar.

Table 2. Farm level *Brucella* seroprevalence (95% confidence interval) in the five different cities.

	Brucella **Farm Positivity**	*Brucella* **Farm Positivity Excluding Farms with Vaccination**
Bangalore	2.9% (0.6–8.4)	3.0% (0.6–8.6)
Bhubaneswar	2.0% (0.2–6.9)	1.4% (0–7.4)
Guwahati	73.5% (63.9–81.8)	72.5% (62.5–81.0)
Ludhiana	4.9% (1.6–11.1)	4.3% (1.2–10.6)
Udaipur	5.9% (2.2–12.4)	5.2% (1.7–11.6)
Overall	17.8% (14.6–21.34)	18.3% (14.8–22.1)

3.2. Risk Factor Analyses for Herds with No Previous Vaccination

The presence of different stipulated risk factors varied across the five cities. After exclusion of farms that reported having vaccinated against *Brucella* earlier, 460 farms from 162 villages in five sites (geographic regions) were included. Missing values were observed in 0 to 15.6% of observations within a variable and 62% of farms had complete data for all variables. *Brucella* prevalence ranged from 1.4 to 5.2% across four sites, while the prevalence in Guwahati was 72.5%.

The MCA analysis for investigating relationships among predictors identified pasture grazing, use of artificial insemination (AI) (vs natural breeding), routine (vs irregular) vaccination, floor cleanliness, adequacy of floor drainage, and owner knowledge of antibiotics as the six variables most useful in discriminating among farms. Floor cleanliness and drainage contributed most to the first dimension (explaining 51.3% of inertia (information) in the data) while level of vaccination, knowledge of antibiotics and AI contributed most to the second dimension (45.0% of inertia). Farmers that had knowledge of antibiotics also used routine vaccination, and they tended to be farms that did not pasture (graze) animals but did use AI. Farms with good floor cleanliness also had good floor drainage.

Evaluation of unconditional associations between the recorded predictors and Guwahati vs the other sites showed many statistically significant differences. With the exception of three of the four demographic variables and the quarantining of new entries into the herd, all predictors showed significant differences at $p < 0.05$. Compared to the other cities, Guwahati had larger non-pastured herds, used AI for breeding, purchased their replacements from neighbors, were less likely to have good stable cleanliness or drainage scores, were more likely to have dirty stable floors, had a lower composite hygiene score, and were less likely to have veterinarians regularly check their animals or check animals before purchase. However, they were more likely to use routine vaccinations of young animals and to know what antibiotics were.

3.3. Risk Factors for Brucella Seropositivity in Guwahati

In addition to age and herd size, which were included as potential confounders, two management factors (floor cleanliness and level of vaccine use) were identified as being associated with *Brucella* spp. A multiple correspondence analysis (MCA) plot was generated (using trichotomous versions of each of the predictors) with *Brucella* spp. added as a supplemental variable to the final plot to see which predictors were generally associated with being *Brucella* spp. positive or negative (Figure 3). Being *Brucella* positive (B1) was most common in farms that had a younger age owner (ag0 or ag1) and had a lower floor cleanliness scores (fc1 or fc2). Being *Brucella* negative (B0) was most strongly associated with the cleanest floors (fc3) and the smallest herds (na0). Table 3 shows the odds ratios associated with seropositivity for risk factors in Guwahati from the multivariable model. The high village level variance indicates a very high intra-cluster correlation.

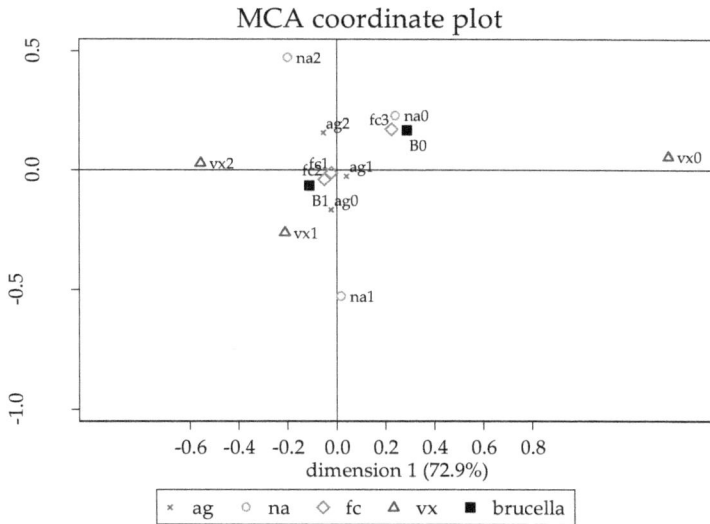

Figure 3. MCA plot of risk factors for *Brucella* seropositivity in Guwahati, India. Ai = Artificial insemination, where ai0 is no artificial insemination and ai1 is use of artificial insemination. Na = number of animals, where na0 is less than 7 animals and na1 is 7–10 animals. Fc = floor cleanliness, where fc0 is clean or moderately clean floor and fc1 is dirty floor. Vx = vaccination, where vx0 means no vaccination done, vx1 means vaccination when there is an outbreak or when given free vaccines, and vx2 means vaccinating animals as young. B = *Brucella*, where B0 = seronegative farm and B1 = seropositive farm.

Table 3. Risk factors for *Brucella* seropositivity within Guwahati, India, using a mixed logistic regression model.

Risk Factor	Odds Ratio	95% Confidence Interval	Standard Error	*p*-Value
Farmer age (year)	0.96	0.90–1.02	0.03	0.20
Floor cleanliness				
Clean	Reference			
Average	11.6	1.29–105.18	13.1	0.03
Dirty	42.8	1.87–978.57	68.3	0.02
Vaccination				
No vaccination	Reference			
Vaccinate irregularly	44.1	0.73–2669.57	92.3	0.07
Vaccinate routinely	12.8	1.40–116.80	14.4	0.02
Number of animals	1.0	0.85–1.30	0.4	0.7
Quadratic term of number of animals	0.95	0.90–0.999	0.02	0.05
Constant	2.2	0.05–91.5	4.1	
Village level variance	4.2	0.65–26.84	4.0	

3.4. Risk Factors for Brucella Seropositivity in Bangalore, Bhubaneswar, Ludhiana, and Udaipur

Logistic models were also used to investigate risk factors for *Brucella* spp. positivity within the low-prevalence sites. However, no risk factors had significant associations, so no results are presented.

4. Discussion

This study found high variation in the seroprevalence between the different peri-urban sites. In general, our findings were comparable with the literature on bovine brucellosis in India. A recent review concluded that most studies using probabilistic sampling and not targeting cows with a clinical history suggesting brucellosis, reported a prevalence of 5–12%, which is above what was detected in the four other cities but considerably less than that we found in Guwahati [20]. While this study could not identify many risk factors in the peri-urban farms, it was found that keeping floors clean was important. Risk of *Brucella* exposure was also associated with herd size, which has been shown previously [21–24]. Vaccinating (for other diseases than brucellosis), either routinely or when there were vaccination campaigns in the face of outbreaks or vaccines provided for free, was associated with a higher risk of exposure, which could potentially be explained as farmers with more experience with disease being more positive to vaccination.

The peri-urban seroprevalence in Ludhiana, Punjab, was lower than previously reported in the state. Here 21% and 18% seroprevalence was found by Aulakh et al. [25] and Ul-Islam et al. [26]. Gill et al. [23] and Dhand et al. [27] also found more than 10% prevalence in cattle. This may indicate that reducing prevalence is associated with better control or changing husbandry, or may reflect a more systematic approach to sampling in our study, which focused only on smallholder peri-urban dairying.

The high seropositivity in Guwahati is in accordance with results from the same area using a milk ring test, where 88% of farms were found positive [28]. Chakraborty et al. [29] found 60% seropositivity among lactating cows in Guwahati, whereas Gogoi et al. [30] found 30% seroprevalence in Kamrup metropolitan district of Guwahati. It is worth noting that Renukaradhya et al. [31] did not find any seropositive animals in Assam, using their own developed ELISA. Given the results of our research and the earlier research from the state, it seems that the peri-urban belt around Guwahati may have a higher than average burden of brucellosis. Brucellosis in humans has not been extensively studied, but in one previous study, three (all with animal husbandry background) out of 52 humans tested positive in Assam [32]. In people with animal contact, more than 24% seropositivity was found in Ludhiana as well [33], indicating the need to include brucellosis as a potential diagnosis in febrile cases with occupational risk factors.

The study shows how MCA can be used when data are collected on quite a large number of predictors and many of these are potentially related (weakly or strongly). In this context, it is useful to visualize these inter-relationships in order to get a better understanding of how farms could be grouped. The MCA identified a set of key variables which could be used to discriminate among farms, and these should be considered as important to collect information on in any future research undertaken in this region of India. Another methodological issue was presented because one site (Guwahati) had an extremely high herd prevalence of *Brucella* spp. compared to the other four sites. The strong collinearity between the outcome of interest (seropositivity against *Brucella*) and the site meant that the risk factor analyses could not utilize the full data set in one analysis. It would have been impossible to tell if any significant predictor was actually associated with *Brucella* spp. positivity or whether it just strongly differed between Guwahati and the other sites (with no effect on *Brucella* spp. risk). Consequently, risk factors were evaluated in Guwahati separately from the other study sites, which reduced the power of the study. For the four low-prevalence sites, there were only 14 positive farms (out of 362) while in Guwahati there were only 27 negative farms (out of 98). This lack of power limited our ability to identify risk factors for *Brucella* spp.

Raising awareness, training farmers, and modern techniques are often recommended for improving livestock disease control. In our study, the evidence for this was ambiguous. Guwahati, which had the highest prevalence in this study, was characterized by greater knowledge and higher use of modern animal health care inputs, such as vaccination and AI. On the other hand, hygiene appeared to be poor. Overall, a picture emerges of larger, less well managed herds with more reliance on vaccines and antibiotics for disease control. Other studies in Guwahati found that while training interventions had some impact on both hygiene and knowledge, there was no impact on the seropositivity for brucellosis [28]. This indicates caution in assuming intensification, even with improving knowledge and training, will lead to better disease control. It should be noted, however, that overall use of vaccination was low, indicating considerable scope for improvement. There seemed to be a high dependency on vaccinations in the face of outbreaks or when they were provided for free, with two of the sites having less than 3% of farms reporting routine vaccinations. Poor vaccination coverage can have different explanations, including poor access to vaccines, limited extension services, or poor understanding of farmers as to the benefits of using vaccines. In other studies in India, low knowledge about the function of vaccines and low willingness to pay has been associated with low uptake of vaccination [34,35], which could possibly also explain the low adoption here. Studying the use of vaccines in chickens, it has been shown that having active support promotes vaccination and also makes people understand the function of vaccines better, which makes for more positive attitudes, and hence better uptake [36]. Even though farms that reported having used *Brucella* vaccines were excluded from analyses, it is possible that there might be farms where the farmer did not know which disease the animals were vaccinated against, which could have affected the results, but considering the low vaccination against *Brucella* overall, this is deemed a low risk. India has a government sponsored control program for brucellosis in cattle, with planned use of the S19 vaccine [31], but still vaccination is seldom performed in the field.

Many sero-surveys have been carried out for brucellosis in India, but these are typically conducted in one area, and differing methods make it hard to compare results from different areas, including the frequent targeting of animals with clinical symptoms [20]. Using the same, probabilistic study approach contemporaneously in five widely dispersed cities allowed us to confidently detect important and likely real differences between cities and to link this with some risk factors. An important finding of the study was that brucellosis can be very prevalent in some peri-urban areas and have very low presence in others. Moreover, disease transmission risk factors are different in scenarios with a high or a low infection pressure, and a habit, such as purchasing cows from neighbors is likely a protective factor when living in a low-risk area, but a high-risk practice in an area with a very high prevalence. Within Guwahati, the mixed effects model suggested a very high village level variance and a high intra-cluster correlation, indicating that future studies need to include as many villages as possible, which could be explained by the habit of purchasing animals from nearby farms, spreading the disease within a village, but less so between villages.

5. Conclusions

This study emphasizes the need to systematically identify disease hotspots for zoonotic diseases; the importance of considering intensifying peri-urban dairy belts in disease surveillance and control; the high degree to which structural factors may influence disease risk in peri-urban dairy, and the need for targeted, effective interventions. In light of the brucellosis control program in India, this study highlights the lack of sufficient vaccination coverage among smallholder dairy farmers in different parts of India, and also the high variability in prevalence. Knowledge about the prevalence in different areas can guide the control efforts, and improved information about local risk factors as well as the extent of farmers' understanding about the disease, can aid in creating better extension campaigns.

Author Contributions: J.F.L., M.K. & D.G. conceptualized and designed the project, J.F.L. & I.D. conducted the data analyses, J.S.B. & J.P.S.G. conducted laboratory analyses, A.S.C., R.A.H., N.M.F. & M.K. coordinated data collection, J.F.L. drafted the manuscript & all authors contributed to critically revise the manuscript.

Funding: This study was part of a larger project supported by International Development Research Centre, Canada grant (No.107344–001). The project was also supported by the CGIAR Research Program for Nutrition and Health.

Acknowledgments: The authors would like to acknowledge all participating farmers, the data collection teams and other collaborators.

Conflicts of Interest: The authors declare no conflict of interest.

References

1.   WHO FAO OIE; Corbel, M.J. *Brucellosis in Humans and Animals*; WHO: Rome, Italy, 2006.
2.   Pappas, G.; Papadimitriou, P.; Akritidis, N.; Christou, L.; Tsianos, E.V. The new global map of human brucellosis. *Lancet. Infect. Dis.* **2006**, *6*, 91–99. [CrossRef]
3.   OIE. *Bovine Brucellosis: OIE Terrestrial Manual 2009*; Office International de Epizootie: Paris, France, 2009.

4. McDermott, J.J.; Grace, D.; Zinsstag, J. Economics of brucellosis impact and control in low-income countries. *Sci. Tech. Rev. Off. Int. Des Epizoot.* **2013**, *32*, 249–261. [CrossRef]

5. Godfroid, J.; Nielsen, K.; Saegerman, C. Diagnosis of brucellosis in livestock and wildlife. *Croat. Med. J.* **2010**, *51*, 296–305. [CrossRef] [PubMed]

6. OIE. Infection with Brucella abortus, Brucella melitensis and Brucella suis. In *OIE Terrestrial Manual 2016*; OIE (World Organisation for Animal Health): Rome, Italy, 2016.

7. Seleem, M.N.; Boyle, S.M.; Sriranganathan, N. Brucellosis: A re-emerging zoonosis. *Vet. Microbiol.* **2010**, *140*, 392–398. [CrossRef] [PubMed]

8. Millar, M.; Stack, J. Brucellosis—What every practitioner should know. *Practice* **2012**, *34*, 532–539. [CrossRef]

9. Delgado, C.L. Rising Consumption of Meat and Milk in Developing Countries Has Created a New Food Revolution. *J. Nutr.* **2003**, *133*, 3907S–3910S. [CrossRef]

10. FAOSTAT. Milk Total Production in India. 2015. Available online: http://faostat3.fao.org/browse/Q/QL/E (accessed on 12 April 2015).

11. Douphrate, D.I.; Hagevoort, G.R.; Nonnenmann, M.W.; Lunner Kolstrup, C.; Reynolds, S.J.; Jakob, M.; Kinsel, M. The dairy industry: A brief description of production practices, trends, and farm characteristics around the world. *J. Agromed.* **2013**, *18*, 187–197. [CrossRef] [PubMed]

12. Thumbi, S.M.; Njenga, M.K.; Marsh, T.L.; Noh, S.; Otiang, E.; Munyua, P.; Ochieng, L.; Ogola, E.; Yoder, J.; Audi, A.; et al. Linking Human Health and Livestock Health: A "One-Health" Platform for Integrated Analysis of Human Health, Livestock Health, and Economic Welfare in Livestock Dependent Communities. *PLoS ONE* **2015**, *10*, e0120761. [CrossRef]

13. Grace, D.; Wanyoike, F.; Lindahl, J.; Bett, B.; Randolph, T.; Rich, K.M. Poor livestock keepers: Ecosystem-poverty-health interactions. *Philos. Trans. R. Soc. B-Econ.* **2017**, *372*, 20160166. [CrossRef]

14. Omemo, P.; Ogola, E.; Omondi, G.; Wasonga, J.; Knobel, D. Knowledge, attitude and practice towards zoonoses among public health workers in Nyanza province, Kenya. *J. Public Health Afr.* **2012**, *3*, 22. [CrossRef]

15. de Glanville, W.A.; Conde-Álvarez, R.; Moriyón, I.; Njeru, J.; Díaz, R.; Cook, E.A.J.; Morin, M.; de, C.; Bronsvoort, B.M.; Thomas, L.F.; Kariuki, S.; et al. Poor performance of the rapid test for human brucellosis in health facilities in Kenya. *PLoS Negl. Trop. Dis.* **2017**, *11*, e0005508. [CrossRef]

16. Lindahl, J.F.; Vrentas, C.E.; Ram, P.; Deka, R.A.; Hazarika, H.; Rahman, R.G.; Bambal, J.S.; Bedi, C.; Pallab Chaduhuri, B.; Fairoze, N.M.; et al. Brucellosis in India: Results of a collaborative workshop to define One Health priorities. *Trop. Anim. Health Prod.* **2019**. (submitted).

17. Lindahl, J.F.; Chauhan, A.; Gill, J.P.S.; Hazarika, R.A.; Fairoze, N.M.; Grace, D.; Kakkar, M. The extent and structure of peri-urban smallholder dairy farming in five cities in India. *Trop. Anim. Health Prod.* **2019**. (submitted).

18. Emmerzaal, A.; de Wit, J.J.; Dijkstra, T.; Bakker, D.; van Zijderveld, F.G. The Dutch *Brucella abortus* monitoring programme for cattle: The impact of false-positive serological reactions and comparison of serological tests. *Vet. Q.* **2002**, *24*, 40–46. [CrossRef] [PubMed]

19. Gall, D.; Nielsen, K. Serological Diagnosis of Bovine Brucellosis: A Review of Test Performance and Cost Comparison. *Rev. sci. tech. Off. int. Epiz.* **2004**, *23*, 3. [CrossRef]

20. Deka, R.P.; Magnusson, U.; Grace, D.; Lindahl, J. Bovine brucellosis: Prevalence, risk factors, economic cost and control options with particular reference to India—A review. *Infect. Ecol. Epidemiol.* **2018**, *8*, 1556548. [CrossRef]

21. Makita, K.; Fèvre, E.M.; Waiswa, C.; Eisler, M.C.; Thrusfield, M.; Welburn, S.C. Herd prevalence of bovine brucellosis and analysis of risk factors in cattle in urban and peri-urban areas of the Kampala economic zone, Uganda. *BMC Vet. Res.* **2011**, *7*, 60. [CrossRef]

22. Mugizi, D.R.; Boqvist, S.; Nasinyama, G.W.; Waiswa, C.; Ikwap, K.; Rock, K.; Lindahl, E.; Magnusson, U.; Erume, J. Prevalence of and factors associated with Brucella sero-positivity in cattle in urban and peri-urban Gulu and Soroti towns of Uganda. *J. Vet. Med. Sci.* **2015**, *77*, 557–564. [CrossRef]

23. Gill, J.; Kaur, S.; Joshi, D.; Sharma, J. Epidemiological studies on brucellosis in farm animals in Punjab state of India and its public health significance. In Proceedings of the 9th International Symposium on Veterinary Epidemiology and Economics, Breckenridge, CO, USA, 6–11 August 2000.

24. Patel, M.; Patel, P.; Prajapati, M.; Kanani, A.N.; Tyagi, K.K.; Fulsoundar, A.B. Prevalence and risk factor's analysis of bovine brucellosis in peri-urban areas under intensive system of production in Gujarat, India. *Vet. World* **2014**, *7*, 509–516. [CrossRef]

25. Aulakh, H.K.; Patil, P.K.; Sharma, S.; Kumar, H.; Mahajan, V.; Sandhu, K.S. A study on the epidemiology of bovine brucellosis in Punjab (India) using milk-ELISA. *Acta Vet. Brno.* **2008**, *77*, 393–399. [CrossRef]
26. Ul-Islam, M.R.; Gupta, M.P.; Filia, G.; Sidhu, P.K.; Shafi, T.A.; Bhat, S.A.; Hussain, S.A.; Mustafa, R.; Verma, A.K.; Sinha, D.K. Sero-epidemiology of brucellosis in organized cattle and buffaloes in Punjab (India). *Adv. Anim. Vet. Sci.* **2013**, *1*, 5–8.
27. Dhand, N.K.; Gumber, S.; Singh, B.B.; Aradhana; Bali, M.S.; Kumar, H.; Sharma, D.R.; Singh, J.; Sandhu, K.S. A study on the epidemiology of brucellosis in Punjab (India) using Survey Toolbox. *Rev. Sci. Tech.* **2005**, *24*, 879–885. [CrossRef]
28. Lindahl, J.F.; Deka, R.P.; Melin, D.; Berg, A.; Lundén, H.; Lapar, M.L.; Asse, R.; Grace, D. An inclusive and participatory approach to changing policies and practices for improved milk safety in Assam, northeast India. *Glob. Food Sec.* **2018**, *17*, 9–13. [CrossRef]
29. Chakraborty, M.; Patgiri, G.P.; Barman, N.N. Application of delayed-type hypersensitivity test (DTH) for the diagnosis of bovine brucellosis. *Indian Vet. J.* **2000**, *77*, 849–851.
30. Gogoi, S.B.; Hussain, P.; Sarma, P.C.; Barua, A.G.; Mahato, G.; Bora, D.P.; Konch, P.; Gogoi, P. Prevalence of bovine brucellosis in Assam, India. *J. Entomol. Zool. Stud.* **2017**, *5*, 179–185.
31. Renukaradhya, G.; Isloor, S.; Rajasekhar, M. Epidemiology, zoonotic aspects, vaccination and control/eradication of brucellosis in India. *Vet. Microbiol.* **2002**, *90*, 183–195. [CrossRef]
32. Hussain, S.A.; Rahman, H.; Pal, D.; Ahmed, K. Sero-prevalence of bovine and human brucellosis in Assam. *Indianj. Comp. Microbiol. Immunol. Infect. Dis.* **2000**, *21*, 165–166.
33. Yohannes Gemechu, M.; Paul Singh Gill, J. Seroepidemiological survey of human brucellosis in and around Ludhiana, India. *Emerg. Health Threat. J.* **2011**, *4*, 1–7. [CrossRef]
34. Heffernan, C.; Thomson, K.; Nielsen, L. Caste, livelihoods and livestock: An exploration of the uptake of livestock vaccination adoption among poor farmers in India. *J. Int. Dev.* **2011**, *23*, 103–118. [CrossRef]
35. Basunathe, V.K.; Sawarkar, S.W.; Sasidhar, P.V.K. Adoption of Dairy Production Technologies and Implications for Dairy Development in India. *Outlook Agric.* **2010**, *39*, 134–140. [CrossRef]
36. Lindahl, J.F.; Young, J.; Wyatt, A.; Young, M.; Alders, R.; Bagnol, B.; Kibaya, A.; Grace, D. Do vaccination interventions have effects? A study on how poultry vaccination interventions change smallholder farmer knowledge, attitudes, and practice in villages in Kenya and Tanzania. *Trop. Anim. Health Prod.* **2018**, *51*, 213–220. [CrossRef] [PubMed]

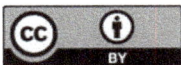

Tropical Medicine and
Infectious Disease

MDPI

Review

Clostridium difficile in Asia: Opportunities for One Health Management

Deirdre A. Collins [1] and **Thomas V. Riley** [1,2,3,*]

1   School of Medical & Health Sciences, Edith Cowan University, Joondalup 6027, Australia;
     deirdre.collins@ecu.edu.au
2   Department of Microbiology, PathWest Laboratory Medicine, Nedlands 6009, Australia
3   School of Veterinary & Life Sciences, Murdoch University, Murdoch 6150, Australia
*   Correspondence: thomas.riley@uwa.edu.au; Tel.: +61-8-6457-3690

Received: 4 December 2018; Accepted: 23 December 2018; Published: 28 December 2018

Abstract: *Clostridium difficile* is a ubiquitous spore-forming bacterium which causes toxin-mediated diarrhoea and colitis in people whose gut microflora has been depleted by antimicrobial use, so it is a predominantly healthcare-associated disease. However, there are many One Health implications to *C. difficile*, given high colonisation rates in food production animals, contamination of outdoor environments by use of contaminated animal manure, increasing incidence of community-associated *C. difficile* infection (CDI), and demonstration of clonal groups of *C. difficile* shared between human clinical cases and food animals. In Asia, the epidemiology of CDI is not well understood given poor testing practices in many countries. The growing middle-class populations of Asia are presenting increasing demands for meat, thus production farming, particularly of pigs, chicken and cattle, is rapidly expanding in Asian countries. Few reports on *C. difficile* colonisation among production animals in Asia exist, but those that do show high prevalence rates, and possible importation of European strains of *C. difficile* like ribotype 078. This review summarises our current understanding of the One Health aspects of the epidemiology of CDI in Asia.

Keywords: *Clostridium difficile*; Asia; epidemiology; One Health

---

1. Introduction

Clostridium difficile is a ubiquitous spore-forming anaerobic bacterium which colonises the infant mammalian and avian gastrointestinal tract before the gut microflora has been established [1]. This "virgin" gut environment is replicated in mammals of all ages during and after antimicrobial exposure, or because of other circumstances that deplete or change the gut microflora. While human infants may not yet express the receptor for *C. difficile* toxins [2], older children and adults who become infected with toxigenic *C. difficile* can experience toxin-mediated disease ranging from self-limiting diarrhoea to life-threatening pseudomembranous colitis (PMC) and/or toxic megacolon.

C. difficile infection (CDI) has been predominantly a healthcare-associated illness, with the majority of cases being of advanced age, with comorbidities and a history of recent hospitalisation or treatment for illness. Increasing reported incidence rates in many regions [3] can partly be explained by the adoption of highly sensitive PCR testing [4] over the past decade, however, rates of community-associated (CA)-CDI are also rising [5,6]. While *C. difficile* spores can survive for long periods of time in healthcare environments due to their resistance to many disinfectants, recent advances in whole genome sequencing (WGS) studies have shown that up to 50% of CDI cases may be acquired from sources outside of healthcare facilities [7], implying environmental exposure accounts for a considerable proportion of CDI cases. High rates of *C. difficile* colonisation among food production livestock in which antimicrobials are frequently overused [8] have increased the risk of zoonotic transmission of *C. difficile* to humans [1]. Studies show high prevalence of *C. difficile* contamination of outdoor environments [9,10] and root vegetables [11] due to the use of contaminated animal manure as fertiliser. WGS has identified clonal groups of *C. difficile* isolated from both humans and animals [12], further supporting the possibility of zoonotic transmission of *C. difficile* from production animals to humans.

Intercontinental epidemics of CDI demonstrate the potential for international spread of *C. difficile*. Examples include the severe outbreaks in North America and Europe caused by clonal strains of ribotype (RT) 027 *C. difficile* originating in North America [13], and outbreaks of clindamycin-resistant strains of RT 017 across Asia, Europe and North America [14–17]. CDI epidemiology has been well documented in North America, Europe and, to a lesser extent, in Australia [5,6,18,19]. Different molecular types of *C. difficile* circulate in these respective regions, primarily ribotype (RT) 027 in North America and, until recently, Europe [20,21], and RT 014/020 in Australia [22]. To date, CDI has been largely under-diagnosed, under-reported and under-investigated in Asia, despite being home to 60% of the world's population, due to poor awareness among physicians and often inappropriate testing [23].

Over recent decades, growing economies and expanding populations across Asia have led to a rising middle class and ageing population with increasing demands for medical and aged care facilities. This wealth increase has also led to a greater appetite for meat and meat products, which has triggered a massive increase in meat consumption [24] and huge population expansion among meat production livestock, most notably pigs, chicken and cattle. This large-scale production farming, growing populations accessing healthcare facilities and widespread overuse of antimicrobials [25] make Asia an environment which is highly conducive to transmission of *C. difficile*, among both humans and animals.

The One Health paradigm approaches public health from a collaborative, multi-sectorial point of view, aiming to integrate policies, legislation and research to achieve better public health outcomes. It is particularly relevant to biosecurity, encompassing zoonotic infection, the rise of antimicrobial resistance and food safety. Given widespread colonisation of production animals and environmental contamination with *C. difficile* spores, management and control of CDI should use a One Health-based approach. This review examines our current knowledge of *C. difficile* in Asia from a One Health perspective.

2. Epidemiology of CDI in Asia

2.1. Diagnostic Practices in Asia

The prevalence and incidence rates of CDI can vary widely according to the testing method used. Diagnostic assays range from enzyme immunoassays (EIAs) detecting glutamate dehydrogenase (GDH) and/or toxin (A, B or both) to PCR for the *tcdA* or *tcdB* genes, to traditional culture and cell culture cytotoxicity assay (CCCA). No diagnostic test besides CCCA is suitable as a stand-alone test since toxin EIAs have low sensitivity, and PCR, GDH EIA and culture cannot rule out cases of transient colonisation [26]. CCCA is laborious and time-consuming so it is not routinely employed in diagnostic settings. Reports from Asia have indicated inappropriate testing in the past, particularly use of toxin A EIAs, which will underdiagnose CDI in Asia due to the high prevalence of toxin A-negative/toxin B-positive (A-B+) RT 017 and RT 369 strains [23]. According to a systematic review of studies in Asia, the most commonly performed tests were culture (71%) followed by EIA (52%) and PCR (51%) [27].

2.2. Estimated Prevalence and Incidence of CDI in Asia

Culture and PCR identify toxigenic *C. difficile* at high prevalence ranging from 9%–11% [28–30] in South-East Asia, while toxin EIA was positive in only 3%–5% of the same study specimens [28,29]. A systematic review of studies of CDI from Asia found a mean overall prevalence of 14.8% among hospital inpatients and outpatients, varying significantly from 2.0% to 61.4% across studies, and

16.4% among hospitalised patients with diarrhoea. The pooled incidence rate of CDI in Asia was calculated by meta-analysis at 5.3/10,000 patient days (95% CI 4.0–6.7) [27]. The random effects pooled CDI-related death rate was estimated at 8.9% (95% CI 5.4%–12.3%) by meta-analysis of existing studies [27], while a 13-country descriptive study with 600 recruited CDI cases found a lower mortality rate of 5.2% [31].

Studies in Singapore have demonstrated how changing testing practices have affected incidence rates. The incidence of CDI in Singapore was reported as increasing during the early 2000s, and from 2001 to 2006 the number of samples tested each year increased from 906 to 3508, with the percentage of positive samples increasing from 7% to 11% over the same period [32]. Subsequently, the incidence rate appeared to reduce, which was due to continuing increases in the number of samples being tested (4348 in 2006 to 6738 in 2008 between two hospitals) [33]. This suggests that increasing awareness and vigilance among physicians for possible cases of CDI led to more extensive testing among patients with diarrhoeal disease. Limited resources in some settings have resulted in still inadequate or no testing for CDI. For example, in a study in the Philippines, patients with CDI were frequently misdiagnosed with amoebiasis according to endoscopic detection of colitis [34].

2.3. Burden of CDI in Asia

Despite a high prevalence of *C. difficile* in Asia [27,28,30,35], reports of severe outcomes of CDI are rare. Few reports of PMC and toxic megacolon exist from Asian countries [36–43], suggesting they may be less commonly seen than in other regions. Where reports do appear, they are frequently associated with infection with A-B+ strains [36,40]. Recurrence rates are also lower at 9%–13% [31,44–46] than those reported from North America (15%–20%) [6] and Europe (16%–22%) [19,47], however definitions of recurrence can vary from 8 weeks to 90 days for reappearance of symptoms after resolution of disease. The apparent rarity of severe outcomes of CDI in the region, such as PMC or toxic megacolon, is likely influenced by the poor awareness of CDI among physicians. As demonstrated in the study in the Philippines, CDI is misdiagnosed as amoebiasis and treated with metronidazole which is often sufficient for resolution of milder cases of CDI, resulting in missed cases [34].

2.4. Molecular Epidemiology of CDI in Asia

2.4.1. A-B+ C. *difficile* Strains

The most commonly used molecular typing methods for *C. difficile* are PCR ribotyping and multi-locus sequence typing (MLST). Phylogenetic analyses based on MLST describe at least five major population clades of *C. difficile* [48]. As mentioned before, RT 017/ST37, a clade 4 strain [49], is A-B+ [48] and the predominant strain identified in Asia [23,27,28,35,50]. In China, Korea, Indonesia and Malaysia, RT 017 is generally the most common *C. difficile* strain in circulation, and it is also prevalent in Japan (referred to in older papers as ribotype "fr"), Taiwan, Hong Kong, Thailand and Singapore [28–30,51–56]. Exposure to antineoplastic agents, use of nasal feeding tubes and care in one particular hospital ward were associated with infection with RT 017 strains in a hospital in Japan [57]. *C. difficile* RT 017 has also caused major outbreaks of CDI outside of Asia, in Canada [58] and Europe [15,16], and is frequently reported as having enhanced fluoroquinolone and clindamycin resistance [15,16], a feature that has most likely contributed to its success as an epidemic strain.

The emergence of *C. difficile* RT 369/ST81, another clade 4 A-B+ strain, is also of interest and warrants close monitoring [31,59,60]. This strain apparently emerged first in Japan, where historically it was referred to in the literature using local nomenclature as "trf" [60,61]. It appears that RT 369 caused outbreaks of CDI in hospitals in 2000 and 2001, when ribotyping was not performed [57,60,62]. The first report of RT 369 was in a study conducted on isolates collected from outbreak and non-outbreak situations from 2009–2013 in Japan. This study detected RT 369 in an outbreak setting in a hospital in 2009 [60], and it is now one of the most common strains in circulation there [31,59]. RT 369 has since been reported in studies from China as the cause of a nosocomial outbreak among hospital patients in

Shanghai in 2014 and 2015 where it was the most common strain in circulation. RT 369/ST81 strains are also reported to have higher rates of resistance to clindamycin, ciprofloxacin and moxifloxacin compared with other strains, and a higher sporulation rate than RT 017/ST37 strains [63,64].

2.4.2. Binary Toxin-Positive *C. difficile* Strains

Many but not all binary toxin-positive (CDT+) *C. difficile* strains tend to group in phylogenetic clades 2 and 5, and have been associated with epidemics of CDI in North America (RT 027/ST1, clade 2) [13,65], Europe (RT 078/ST11, clade 5, and RT 027/ST1) [19,21] and Australia (RT 244/ST41, clade 2) [66] in recent times. In contrast, CDT+ strains have been only sporadically reported from Asia and major epidemics like those seen elsewhere have not occurred [67]. Most cases of RT 027 infection to date have been reported from China, where 11 cases were reported from one hospital over 3 years [68]. RT 027 also caused CDI among seven patients across four hospitals in Seoul and Gyenngi province in Korea [69], and may be increasing in prevalence in Taiwan, where it was never reported prior to 2015 [70,71]. Most Asian RT 027 *C. difficile* strains investigated to date have not been related to either of the two main epidemic RT 027 lineages referred to as FQR1 and FQR2 [13], and many have been reported as fluoroquinolone-susceptible, unlike the epidemic lineages.

C. difficile RT 078 (CDT+) was reported among eight cases of CDI across three hospitals in China, where it was also isolated from environmental surfaces suggesting nosocomial transmission [72]. RT 078-related strains RT 126 and 127 (both ST11) are more common in Taiwan, where they were the most common CDT+ strains reported from Southern Taiwan between 2011 and 2013 [73]. A subsequent nationwide study from 2015–2016 identified RTs 078, 126 and 127 at significant prevalence among 842 toxigenic isolates (1.5%, 3.1% and 2.9%, respectively), mainly confined to two hospitals [70].

2.4.3. A+B+ *C. difficile* Strains

C. difficile clade 1 strains that are mainly A+B+ are also frequently reported from Asia. RT 018/ST17 is the predominant clade 1 strain found in the region with the earliest reports coming from Japan (referred to as ribotype "smz") [23]. A closely related strain, "smz'"/QX 239/ST17 is now also circulating at high prevalence in Japan [59,60]. RT 018 is now the most common *C. difficile* strain reported from Korea, where it has largely replaced RT 017 [23,74]. RT 012/ST54 and RT 046/ST35 localise to China in particular [75–79], RT 014/020/ST2/14 is widespread across the continent [31], and RT 002/ST8 is most frequently reported from Taiwan and Hong Kong [31,80].

2.4.4. Non-Toxigenic *C. difficile* Strains

A notable aspect of the molecular epidemiology of *C. difficile* in Asia is the high prevalence of non-toxigenic strains, particularly in South-East Asia. In recent studies in Thailand, Indonesia and Malaysia [28,30,35], non-toxigenic strains of *C. difficile*, most commonly RTs 009 and 010, QX 083, QX 002 and QX 083, were isolated at a prevalence of 50% among all study isolates. Further north in Asia, non-toxigenic strains are reported less frequently (24%, Taiwan [70] 8%–11%, China [76,79,81]), however, this may be a reflection of the use of diagnostic methods other than culture, which would not detect non-toxigenic strains. These strains are incapable of causing CDI but can colonise the gut when the normal flora are disrupted due to antimicrobial use. Many group in the predominantly non-toxigenic MLST clade 4 [49]. The high prevalence of RT 017 and non-toxigenic strains [28,30,35] suggests that clade 4 may have evolved in the Asian region, but further studies on non-toxigenic strains both in Asia and elsewhere are required to determine whether this is the case.

The unique molecular epidemiology of *C. difficile* in Asia (described in more detail in Collins et al. [23]), particularly the high prevalence of non-toxigenic strains, likely plays a role in the overall apparently less severe manifestations of disease seen in the region. Therapeutic administration of non-toxigenic *C. difficile* can protect against recurrent CDI [82], which occurs more rarely among Asian patients (9.1% of cases) than elsewhere [31]. Thus, it is highly plausible that the high prevalence of non-toxigenic strains is protective against recurrence and possibly reduces risk of exposure to virulent strains in Asia. However, many non-toxigenic Asian *C. difficile* strains are resistant to multiple antimicrobials, possibly due to inappropriate antimicrobial use in the region, and they may pose a risk in terms of transmission of antimicrobial resistance (AMR) genes. There have been concerning, albeit rare, reports of metronidazole-resistant non-toxigenic strains [79,83], which should be closely monitored in the region.

3. Prevalence and Molecular Epidemiology of *C. difficile* among Production Animals in Asia

3.1. Prevalence of C. difficile Colonisation and Strain Types in Asian Production Animals

While there are few reports on *C. difficile* in animals in Asia, the prevalence appears to be high among production swine across the continent. A study of 120 neonatal piglets in Japan found a prevalence of *C. difficile* of 57.5%; 61.0% of strains were toxigenic [84]. A high prevalence of 19.3% among 910 pigs of all ages across 47 farms has been reported in Korea, with peak prevalence in diarrheic suckling piglets (53.6%) followed by diarrheic sows (40.0%); again, the majority of isolates (86.9%) was toxigenic [85]. In Taiwan, the prevalence of *C. difficile* among 204 pigs on 13 commercial farms was 49% [86]. The only report to date of *C. difficile* among production animals in South-East Asia comes from Thailand, where the prevalence of *C. difficile* was 35% among piglets (*n* = 165), with all 58 isolates reported as non-toxigenic [87]. RT 078 and closely-related strains including RTs 126 and 127 are the most commonly reported toxigenic strains in pigs in Korea (RT 078 86.5%, RT 126 13.5% of toxigenic strains) [85], Taiwan (RT 078 18%, RT 126 28%, RT 127 43% of toxigenic strains) [86] and Japan (RT 078 third most common strain; 19.7% of toxigenic strains) [84], countries where demand for pork and pork products has surged in recent decades.

3.2. Possible International Sources of C. difficile among Asian Production Animals

To date, *C. difficile* RT 078 and related strains RT 126 and 127 have rarely infected humans in Asia apart from in Taiwan [70,73,88] and, given the apparent endemicity of RT 078 among production animals and human infections in mainland Europe and North America, it is plausible that the strain was introduced into northern Asia via live animal imports. Supporting evidence has been reported from Japan; multi-locus variable number tandem repeat analysis (MLVA) found that Japanese piglet isolates clustered with European human and pig RT 078 strains, giving a strong likelihood that they were imported into Japan from Europe via live breeding pig imports [84]. Live breeding pigs and cattle are imported from Europe, Australia and North America to many Asian countries including Japan [89], China, Taiwan, Vietnam, Cambodia, Malaysia and Thailand (ahdb.org.uk). RTs 078 and 127 are common among cattle and pigs in Europe [90] and RTs 126 and 127 are frequently reported in cattle in Australia [91].

C. difficile RT 078 has also been reported in thoroughbred racehorses, which are frequently traded internationally, in Japan. Five cases of postoperative colitis were documented from the same facility, indicating contamination with a single clone [92]. Further analysis using WGS of RT 078 strains from Japanese racehorses identified a sub-lineage associated with a nosocomial outbreak. RT 027 and RT 017 were also reported, with high relatedness to several reported European strains including clinical isolates from Ireland [93], a prolific producer of racehorses.

4. Discussion

4.1. Systematic Testing Is Required to Identify True CDI Cases in Asia

Introduction of systematic, comprehensive testing for CDI across Asia could provide a better understanding of the epidemiology of CDI in the region, particularly accurate measurement of incidence and prevalence, and deepen our understanding of the burden of CDI. While there is still considerable international debate about optimal testing practices for CDI, colonisation rates with both toxigenic and non-toxigenic *C. difficile* among hospital inpatients are particularly high in

South-East Asia. Many Asian countries are popular destinations for "medical tourism" and there is a risk of transmission of strains via medical tourists returning to their own countries after their treatment. Due to the high prevalence of colonization, it is important to use a diagnostic test which will discriminate true cases of CDI from cases of colonization. GDH and toxin EIA can be performed at relatively low cost and will identify most cases of true infection, despite its lower sensitivity, so it may be the best choice currently for Asian laboratories in developing countries.

Given the apparently uniquely high prevalence of non-toxigenic *C. difficile* strains in Asia, particularly in South-East Asia, it is important to monitor colonization as well. The high prevalence suggests that hospital environments may be heavily contaminated due to poor cleaning or hand hygiene, which puts vulnerable patients at higher risk of CDI. Monitoring of *C. difficile* colonization would also allow further investigation of whether non-toxigenic *C. difficile* colonization is protecting Asian patients from developing CDI and reducing their risk of recurrent disease.

4.2. One Health Implications of CDI in Asia

4.2.1. C. difficile in Asian Production Animals Warrants Close Observation

While there are still relatively few reports of *C. difficile* among Asian production animals, and no reports yet of environmental contamination, the prevalence of *C. difficile* among pigs across Asia is markedly high. Given the significantly increasing demands for pork and pork products, particularly in China and Taiwan, biosecurity measures to ensure these meat products do not pose a threat to humans should include monitoring for *C. difficile* contamination. A spatial epidemiology study in the USA identified increased risk of CA-CDI among people living close to livestock farms [94]. China currently holds half the world's pig population in addition to being the most populated country in the world, so there is a significant risk of infection of a substantial population. In Taiwan, the presence of "hypervirulent" RT 078 and related strains among pigs and increasing prevalence of these strains among clinical cases of CDI suggests transmission of strains between pigs and humans has already occurred. This could be confirmed using WGS studies, as described in an Australian study showing clonal relationships between *C. difficile* isolates from human clinical cases and pigs located thousands of kilometres apart [12].

4.2.2. Live Animal Imports and Exports: Plausible International Routes of Transmission of C. difficile

Genotypic studies of pig and racehorse *C. difficile* isolates from Japan are showing a possibly significant international transmission route of *C. difficile* via live animal imports and exports. The international live animal trade market is a growing sector. From a One Health perspective, it is most important to monitor animals traded with the intention of farming for meat production, as these are kept in close quarters and are thus frequently prophylactically treated with antimicrobials to reduce risk of infection and loss of stock.

5. Conclusions

A One Health approach will be important in management and control of CDI in Asia. It is most important to establish comprehensive testing policies, to identify the true incidence of CDI in Asia before being able to implement effective control measures.

Funding: This research received no external funding.

Conflicts of Interest: The authors declare no conflict of interest.

References

1. Moono, P.; Foster, N.F.; Hampson, D.J.; Knight, D.R.; Bloomfield, L.E.; Riley, T.V. *Clostridium difficile* infection in production animals and avian species: A review. *Foodborne Pathog. Dis.* **2016**, *13*, 647–655. [CrossRef]

2. Eglow, R.; Pothoulakis, C.; Itzkowitz, S.; Israel, E.J.; O'Keane, C.J.; Gong, D.; Gao, N.; Xu, Y.L.; Walker, W.A.; LaMont, J.T. Diminished *Clostridium difficile* toxin A sensitivity in newborn rabbit ileum is associated with decreased toxin A receptor. *J. Clin. Investig.* **1992**, *90*, 822–829. [CrossRef] [PubMed]

3. Martin, J.S.; Monaghan, T.M.; Wilcox, M.H. *Clostridium difficile* infection: Epidemiology, diagnosis and understanding transmission. *Nat. Rev. Gastroenterol. Hepatol.* **2016**, *13*, 206–216. [CrossRef] [PubMed]

4. Polage, C.R.; Gyorke, C.E.; Kennedy, M.A.; Leslie, J.L.; Chin, D.L.; Wang, S.; Nguyen, H.H.; Huang, B.; Tang, Y.W.; Lee, L.W.; et al. Overdiagnosis of *Clostridium difficile* infection in the molecular test era. *JAMA Intern. Med.* **2015**, *175*, 1792–1801. [CrossRef] [PubMed]

5. Slimings, C.; Armstrong, P.; Beckingham, W.D.; Bull, A.L.; Hall, L.; Kennedy, K.J.; Marquess, J.; McCann, R.; Menzies, A.; Mitchell, B.G.; et al. Increasing incidence of *Clostridium difficile* infection, Australia, 2011–2012. *Med. J. Aust.* **2014**, *200*, 272–276. [CrossRef] [PubMed]

6. Lessa, F.C.; Mu, Y.; Bamberg, W.M.; Beldavs, Z.G.; Dumyati, G.K.; Dunn, J.R.; Farley, M.M.; Holzbauer, S.M.; Meek, J.I.; Phipps, E.C.; et al. Burden of *Clostridium difficile* infection in the United States. *N. Engl. J. Med.* **2015**, *372*, 825–834. [CrossRef] [PubMed]

7. Eyre, D.W.; Cule, M.L.; Wilson, D.J.; Griffiths, D.; Vaughan, A.; O'Connor, L.; Ip, C.L.; Golubchik, T.; Batty, E.M.; Finney, J.M.; et al. Diverse sources of *C. difficile* infection identified on whole-genome sequencing. *N. Engl. J. Med.* **2013**, *369*, 1195–1205. [CrossRef]

8. Van Boeckel, T.P.; Brower, C.; Gilbert, M.; Grenfell, B.T.; Levin, S.A.; Robinson, T.P.; Teillant, A.; Laxminarayan, R. Global trends in antimicrobial use in food animals. *Proc. Natl. Acad. Sci. USA* **2015**, *112*, 5649–5654. [CrossRef]

9. Moono, P.; Lim, S.C.; Riley, T.V. High prevalence of toxigenic *Clostridium difficile* in public space lawns in Western Australia. *Sci. Rep.* **2017**, *7*, 41196. [CrossRef]

10. Lim, S.C.; Androga, G.O.; Knight, D.R.; Moono, P.; Foster, N.F.; Riley, T.V. Antimicrobial susceptibility of *Clostridium difficile* isolated from food and environmental sources in Western Australia. *Int. J. Antimicrob. Agents* **2018**, *52*, 411–415. [CrossRef]

11. Lim, S.C.; Foster, N.F.; Elliott, B.; Riley, T.V. High prevalence of *Clostridium difficile* on retail root vegetables, Western Australia. *J. Appl. Microbiol.* **2018**, *124*, 585–590. [CrossRef] [PubMed]

12. Knight, D.R.; Squire, M.M.; Collins, D.A.; Riley, T.V. Genome analysis of *Clostridium difficile* PCR ribotype 014 lineage in Australian pigs and humans reveals a diverse genetic repertoire and signatures of long-range interspecies transmission. *Front. Microbiol.* **2017**, *7*, 2138. [CrossRef] [PubMed]

13. He, M.; Miyajima, F.; Roberts, P.; Ellison, L.; Pickard, D.J.; Martin, M.J.; Connor, T.R.; Harris, S.R.; Fairley, D.; Bamford, K.B.; et al. Emergence and global spread of epidemic healthcare-associated *Clostridium difficile*. *Nat. Genet.* **2013**, *45*, 109–113. [CrossRef] [PubMed]

14. al-Barrak, A.; Embil, J.; Dyck, B.; Olekson, K.; Nicoll, D.; Alfa, M.; Kabani, A. An outbreak of toxin A negative, toxin B positive *Clostridium difficile*-associated diarrhea in a Canadian tertiary-care hospital. *Can. Commun. Dis. Rep.* **1999**, *25*, 65–69. [PubMed]

15. Kuijper, E.J.; de Weerdt, J.; Kato, H.; Kato, N.; van Dam, A.P.; van der Vorm, E.R.; Weel, J.; van Rheenen, C.; Dankert, J. Nosocomial outbreak of *Clostridium difficile*-associated diarrhoea due to a clindamycin-resistant enterotoxin A-negative strain. *Eur. J. Clin. Microbiol. Infect. Dis.* **2001**, *20*, 528–534. [CrossRef] [PubMed]

16. Drudy, D.; Harnedy, N.; Fanning, S.; Hannan, M.; Kyne, L. Emergence and control of fluoroquinolone-resistant, toxin A-negative, toxin B-positive *Clostridium difficile*. *Infect. Control. Hosp. Epidemiol.* **2007**, *28*, 932–940. [CrossRef]

17. Cairns, M.D.; Preston, M.D.; Hall, C.L.; Gerding, D.N.; Hawkey, P.M.; Kato, H.; Kim, H.; Kuijper, E.J.; Lawley, T.D.; Pituch, H.; et al. Comparative genome analysis and global phylogeny of the toxin variant *Clostridium difficile* PCR ribotype 017 reveals the evolution of two independent sublineages. *J. Clin. Microbiol.* **2017**, *55*, 865–876. [CrossRef]

18. Centers for Disease Control and Prevention (CDC). *Antibiotic Resistance Threats in the United States, 2013*; CDC: Atlanta, GA, USA, 2013.

19. Bauer, M.P.; Notermans, D.W.; van Benthem, B.H.; Brazier, J.S.; Wilcox, M.H.; Rupnik, M.; Monnet, D.L.; van Dissel, J.T.; Kuijper, E.J.; ECDIS Study Group. *Clostridium difficile* infection in Europe: A hospital-based survey. *Lancet* **2011**, *377*, 63–73. [CrossRef]

20. Tickler, I.A.; Goering, R.V.; Whitmore, J.D.; Lynn, A.N.; Persing, D.H.; Tenover, F.C.; Healthcare Associated Infection Consortium. Strain types and antimicrobial resistance patterns of *Clostridium difficile* isolates from the United States, 2011 to 2013. *Antimicrob. Agents Chemother.* **2014**, *58*, 4214–4218. [CrossRef]

21. Freeman, J.; Vernon, J.; Morris, K.; Nicholson, S.; Todhunter, S.; Longshaw, C.; Wilcox, M.H.; Pan-European Longitudinal Surveillance of Antibiotic Resistance among Prevalent *Clostridium difficile* Ribotypes' Study Group. Pan-European longitudinal surveillance of antibiotic resistance among prevalent *Clostridium difficile* ribotypes. *Clin. Microbiol. Infect.* **2015**, *21*, 248.e9–248.e16. [CrossRef]

22. Collins, D.A.; Putsathit, P.; Elliott, B.; Riley, T.V. Laboratory-based surveillance of *Clostridium difficile* strains circulating in the Australian healthcare setting in 2012. *Pathology* **2017**, *49*, 309–313. [CrossRef] [PubMed]

23. Collins, D.A.; Hawkey, P.M.; Riley, T.V. Epidemiology of *Clostridium difficile* infection in Asia. *Antimicrob. Resist. Infect. Control* **2013**, *2*, 21. [CrossRef] [PubMed]

24. Larsen, J. China's Growing Hunger for Meat Shown by Move to Buy Smithfield, World's Leading Pork Producer. In *Data Highlights*; Earth Policy Institute: Washington, DC, USA, 2013.

25. Van Boeckel, T.P.; Gandra, S.; Ashok, A.; Caudron, Q.; Grenfell, B.T.; Levin, S.A.; Laxminarayan, R. Global antibiotic consumption 2000 to 2010: An analysis of national pharmaceutical sales data. *Lancet Infect. Dis.* **2014**, *14*, 742–750. [CrossRef]

26. McDonald, L.C.; Gerding, D.N.; Johnson, S.; Bakken, J.S.; Carroll, K.C.; Coffin, S.E.; Dubberke, E.R.; Garey, K.W.; Gould, C.V.; Kelly, C.; et al. Clinical practice guidelines for *Clostridium difficile* infection in adults and children: 2017 update by the Infectious Diseases Society of America (IDSA) and Society for Healthcare Epidemiology of America (SHEA). *Clin. Infect. Dis.* **2018**, *66*, e1–e48. [CrossRef] [PubMed]

27. Borren, N.Z.; Ghadermarzi, S.; Hutfless, S.; Ananthakrishnan, A.N. The emergence of *Clostridium difficile* infection in Asia: A systematic review and meta-analysis of incidence and impact. *PLoS ONE* **2017**, *12*, e0176797. [CrossRef] [PubMed]

28. Collins, D.A.; Gasem, M.H.; Habibie, T.H.; Arinton, I.G.; Hendriyanto, P.; Hartana, A.P.; Riley, T.V. Prevalence and molecular epidemiology of *Clostridium difficile* infection in Indonesia. *New Microbe New Infect.* **2017**, *18*, 34–37. [CrossRef] [PubMed]

29. Riley, T.V.; Collins, D.A.; Karunakaran, R.; Kahar, M.A.; Adnan, A.; Hassan, S.A.; Zainul, N.H.; Rustam, F.R.M.; Wahab, Z.A.; Ramli, R.; et al. High prevalence of toxigenic and nontoxigenic *Clostridium difficile* strains in Malaysia. *J. Clin. Microbiol.* **2018**, *56*. [CrossRef]

30. Putsathit, P.; Maneerattanaporn, M.; Piewngam, P.; Kiratisin, P.; Riley, T.V. Prevalence and molecular epidemiology of *Clostridium difficile* infection in Thailand. *New Microbe New Infect.* **2017**, *15*, 27–32. [CrossRef]

31. Collins, D.A.; Sohn, K.M.; Wu, Y.; Ouchi, K.; Ishii, Y.; Elliott, B.; Riley, T.V.; Tateda, K.; for the Clostridium difficile Asia Pacific (CDAP) Study Group. Clostridium difficile infection in the Asia-Pacific region. In Proceedings of the 27th European Congress of Clinical Microbiology and Infectious Diseases, Vienna, Austria, 22–25 April 2017.

32. Lim, P.L.; Barkham, T.M.; Ling, L.M.; Dimatatac, F.; Alfred, T.; Ang, B. Increasing incidence of *Clostridium difficile*-associated disease, Singapore. *Emerg. Infect. Dis.* **2008**, *14*, 1487–1489. [CrossRef]

33. Hsu, L.Y.; Tan, T.Y.; Koh, T.H.; Kwa, A.L.; Krishnan, P.; Tee, N.W.; Jureen, R. Decline in *Clostridium difficile*-associated disease rates in Singapore public hospitals, 2006 to 2008. *BMC Res. Notes* **2011**, *4*, 77. [CrossRef]

34. Warren, C.A.; Labio, E.; Destura, R.; Sevilleja, J.E.; Jamias, J.D.; Daez, M.L. *Clostridium difficile* and *Entamoeba histolytica* infections in patients with colitis in the Philippines. *Trans. R. Soc. Trop. Med. Hyg.* **2012**, *106*, 424–428. [CrossRef] [PubMed]

35. Zainul, N.H.; Ma, Z.F.; Besari, A.; Siti Asma, H.; Rahman, R.A.; Collins, D.A.; Hamid, N.; Riley, T.V.; Lee, Y.Y. Prevalence of *Clostridium difficile* infection and colonization in a tertiary hospital and elderly community of North-Eastern Peninsular Malaysia. *Epidemiol. Infect.* **2017**, *145*, 3012–3019. [CrossRef] [PubMed]

36. Shin, B.M.; Kuak, E.Y.; Yoo, S.J.; Shin, W.C.; Yoo, H.M. Emerging toxin A-B+ variant strain of *Clostridium difficile* responsible for pseudomembranous colitis at a tertiary care hospital in Korea. *Diagn. Microbiol. Infect. Dis.* **2008**, *60*, 333–337. [CrossRef] [PubMed]

37. Shin, J.Y.; Ko, E.J.; Lee, S.H.; Shin, J.B.; Kim, S.I.; Kwon, K.S.; Kim, H.G.; Shin, Y.W.; Bang, B.W. Refractory pseudomembranous colitis that was treated successfully with colonoscopic fecal microbial transplantation. *Intest. Res.* **2016**, *14*, 83–88. [CrossRef] [PubMed]

38. Nishimura, S.; Kou, T.; Kato, H.; Watanabe, M.; Uno, S.; Senoh, M.; Fukuda, T.; Hata, A.; Yazumi, S. Fulminant pseudomembranous colitis caused by *Clostridium difficile* PCR ribotype 027 in a healthy young woman in Japan. *J. Infect. Chemother.* **2014**, *20*, 729–731. [CrossRef] [PubMed]

39. Wang, J.; Xiao, Y.; Lin, K.; Song, F.; Ge, T.; Zhang, T. Pediatric severe pseudomembranous enteritis treated with fecal microbiota transplantation in a 13-month-old infant. *Biomed. Rep.* **2015**, *3*, 173–175. [CrossRef] [PubMed]

40. Toyokawa, M.; Ueda, A.; Tsukamoto, H.; Nishi, I.; Horikawa, M.; Sunada, A.; Asari, S. Pseudomembranous colitis caused by toxin A-negative/toxin B-positive variant strain of *Clostridium difficile*. *J. Infect. Chemother.* **2003**, *9*, 351–354. [CrossRef]

41. Chen, T.C.; Lu, P.L.; Lin, W.R.; Lin, C.Y.; Wu, J.Y.; Chen, Y.H. Rifampin-associated pseudomembranous colitis. *Am. J. Med. Sci.* **2009**, *338*, 156–158. [CrossRef]

42. Huang, S.C.; Yang, Y.J.; Lee, C.T. Rectal prolapse in a child: An unusual presentation of *Clostridium difficile*-associated pseudomembranous colitis. *Pediatr. Neonatol.* **2011**, *52*, 110–112. [CrossRef]

43. Shen, B.J.; Lin, S.C.; Shueng, P.W.; Chou, Y.H.; Tseng, L.M.; Hsieh, C.H. Pseudomembranous colitis within radiotherapy field following concurrent chemoradiation therapy: A case report. *Onco Targets Ther.* **2013**, *6*, 25–28. [CrossRef]

44. Ryu, H.S.; Kim, Y.S.; Seo, G.S.; Lee, Y.M.; Choi, S.C. Risk factors for recurrent *Clostridium difficile* infection. *Intest. Res.* **2012**, *10*, 176–182. [CrossRef]

45. Choi, H.K.; Kim, K.H.; Lee, S.H.; Lee, S.J. Risk factors for recurrence of *Clostridium difficile* infection: Effect of vancomycin-resistant Enterococci colonization. *J. Korean Med. Sci.* **2011**, *26*, 859–864. [CrossRef] [PubMed]

46. Ho, J.; Dai, R.Z.W.; Kwong, T.N.Y.; Wang, X.; Zhang, L.; Ip, M.; Chan, R.; Hawkey, P.M.K.; Lam, K.L.Y.; Wong, M.C.S.; et al. Disease burden of *Clostridium difficile* infections in adults, Hong Kong, China, 2006–2014. *Emerg. Infect. Dis.* **2017**, *23*, 1671–1679. [CrossRef] [PubMed]

47. Eyre, D.W.; Walker, A.S.; Wyllie, D.; Dingle, K.E.; Griffiths, D.; Finney, J.; O'Connor, L.; Vaughan, A.; Crook, D.W.; Wilcox, M.H.; et al. Predictors of first recurrence of *Clostridium difficile* infection: Implications for initial management. *Clin. Infect. Dis.* **2012**, *55*, S77–S87. [CrossRef] [PubMed]

48. Dingle, K.E.; Elliott, B.; Robinson, E.; Griffiths, D.; Eyre, D.W.; Stoesser, N.; Vaughan, A.; Golubchik, T.; Fawley, W.N.; Wilcox, M.H.; et al. Evolutionary history of the *Clostridium difficile* pathogenicity locus. *Genome Biol. Evol.* **2014**, *6*, 36–52. [CrossRef] [PubMed]

49. Stabler, R.A.; Dawson, L.F.; Valiente, E.; Cairns, M.D.; Martin, M.J.; Donahue, E.H.; Riley, T.V.; Songer, J.G.; Kuijper, E.J.; Dingle, K.E.; et al. Macro and micro diversity of *Clostridium difficile* isolates from diverse sources and geographical locations. *PLoS ONE* **2012**, *7*, e31559. [CrossRef] [PubMed]

50. Putsathit, P.; Kiratisin, P.; Ngamwongsatit, P.; Riley, T.V. *Clostridium difficile* infection in Thailand. *Int. J. Antimicrob. Agents* **2015**, *45*, 1–7. [CrossRef]

51. Huang, H.; Weintraub, A.; Fang, H.; Wu, S.; Zhang, Y.; Nord, C.E. Antimicrobial susceptibility and heteroresistance in Chinese *Clostridium difficile* strains. *Anaerobe* **2010**, *16*, 633–635. [CrossRef]

52. Kim, H.; Jeong, S.H.; Roh, K.H.; Hong, S.G.; Kim, J.W.; Shin, M.G.; Kim, M.N.; Shin, H.B.; Uh, Y.; Lee, H.; et al. Investigation of toxin gene diversity, molecular epidemiology, and antimicrobial resistance of *Clostridium difficile* isolated from 12 hospitals in South Korea. *Korean J. Lab. Med.* **2010**, *30*, 491–497. [CrossRef]

53. Kim, S.J.; Kim, H.; Seo, Y.; Yong, D.; Jeong, S.H.; Chong, Y.; Lee, K. Molecular characterization of toxin A-negative, toxin B-positive variant strains of *Clostridium difficile* isolated in Korea. *Diagn Microbiol. Infect. Dis.* **2010**, *67*, 198–201. [CrossRef] [PubMed]

54. Huang, H.; Wu, S.; Wang, M.; Zhang, Y.; Fang, H.; Palmgren, A.C.; Weintraub, A.; Nord, C.E. Molecular and clinical characteristics of *Clostridium difficile* infection in a University Hospital in Shanghai, China. *Clin. Infect. Dis.* **2008**, *47*, 1606–1608. [CrossRef] [PubMed]

55. Tan, X.Q.; Verrall, A.J.; Jureen, R.; Riley, T.V.; Collins, D.A.; Lin, R.T.; Balm, M.N.; Chan, D.; Tambyah, P.A. The emergence of community-onset *Clostridium difficile* infection in a tertiary hospital in Singapore: A cause for concern. *Int. J. Antimicrob. Agents* **2014**, *43*, 47–51. [CrossRef] [PubMed]

56. Ngamskulrungroj, P.; Sanmee, S.; Putsathit, P.; Piewngam, P.; Elliott, B.; Riley, T.V.; Kiratisin, P. Molecular epidemiology of *Clostridium difficile* infection in a large teaching hospital in Thailand. *PLoS ONE* **2015**, *10*, e0127026. [CrossRef]

57. Komatsu, M.; Kato, H.; Aihara, M.; Shimakawa, K.; Iwasaki, M.; Nagasaka, Y.; Fukuda, S.; Matsuo, S.; Arakawa, Y.; Watanabe, M.; et al. High frequency of antibiotic-associated diarrhea due to toxin A-negative, toxin B-positive *Clostridium difficile* in a hospital in Japan and risk factors for infection. *Eur. J. Clin. Microbiol. Infect. Dis.* **2003**, *22*, 525–529. [CrossRef] [PubMed]

58. Alfa, M.J.; Kabani, A.; Lyerly, D.; Moncrief, S.; Neville, L.M.; Al-Barrak, A.; Harding, G.K.; Dyck, B.; Olekson, K.; Embil, J.M. Characterization of a toxin A-negative, toxin B-positive strain of *Clostridium difficile* responsible for a nosocomial outbreak of *Clostridium difficile*-associated diarrhea. *J. Clin. Microbiol.* **2000**, *38*, 2706–2714. [PubMed]

59. Mori, N.; Yoshizawa, S.; Saga, T.; Ishii, Y.; Murakami, H.; Iwata, M.; Collins, D.A.; Riley, T.V.; Tateda, K. Incorrect diagnosis of *Clostridium difficile* infection in a university hospital in Japan. *J. Infect. Chemother.* **2015**, *21*, 718–722. [CrossRef] [PubMed]

60. Senoh, M.; Kato, H.; Fukuda, T.; Niikawa, A.; Hori, Y.; Hagiya, H.; Ito, Y.; Miki, H.; Abe, Y.; Furuta, K.; et al. Predominance of PCR-ribotypes, 018 (smz) and 369 (trf) of *Clostridium difficile* in Japan: A potential relationship with other global circulating strains? *J. Med. Microbiol.* **2015**, *64*, 1226–1236. [CrossRef]

61. Iwashima, Y.; Nakamura, A.; Kato, H.; Kato, H.; Wakimoto, Y.; Wakiyama, N.; Kaji, C.; Ueda, R. A retrospective study of the epidemiology of *Clostridium difficile* infection at a university hospital in Japan: Genotypic features of the isolates and clinical characteristics of the patients. *J. Infect. Chemother.* **2010**, *16*, 329–333. [CrossRef]

62. Sato, H.; Kato, H.; Koiwai, K.; Sakai, C. [A nosocomial outbreak of diarrhea caused by toxin A-negative, toxin B-positive *Clostridium difficile* in a cancer center hospital]. *Kansenshogaku Zasshi* **2004**, *78*, 312–319. [CrossRef]

63. Wang, B.; Peng, W.; Zhang, P.; Su, J. The characteristics of *Clostridium difficile* ST81, a new PCR ribotype of toxin A- B+ strain with high-level fluoroquinolones resistance and higher sporulation ability than ST37/PCR ribotype 017. *FEMS Microbiol. Lett.* **2018**, *365*. [CrossRef]

64. Qin, J.; Dai, Y.; Ma, X.; Wang, Y.; Gao, Q.; Lu, H.; Li, T.; Meng, H.; Liu, Q.; Li, M. Nosocomial transmission of *Clostridium difficile* genotype ST81 in a general teaching hospital in China traced by whole genome sequencing. *Sci. Rep.* **2017**, *7*, 9627. [CrossRef] [PubMed]

65. Loo, V.G.; Poirier, L.; Miller, M.A.; Oughton, M.; Libman, M.D.; Michaud, S.; Bourgault, A.M.; Nguyen, T.; Frenette, C.; Kelly, M.; et al. A predominantly clonal multi-institutional outbreak of *Clostridium difficile*-associated diarrhea with high morbidity and mortality. *N. Engl. J. Med.* **2005**, *353*, 2442–2449. [CrossRef]

66. Eyre, D.W.; Tracey, L.; Elliott, B.; Slimings, C.; Huntington, P.G.; Stuart, R.L.; Korman, T.M.; Kotsiou, G.; McCann, R.; Griffiths, D.; et al. Emergence and spread of predominantly community-onset *Clostridium difficile* PCR ribotype 244 infection in Australia, 2010 to 2012. *Euro Surveill.* **2015**, *20*, 21059. [CrossRef] [PubMed]

67. Collins, D.A.; Riley, T.V. *Clostridium difficile* guidelines. *Clin. Infect. Dis.* **2018**, *67*, 1639. [CrossRef]

68. Jia, H.; Du, P.; Yang, H.; Zhang, Y.; Wang, J.; Zhang, W.; Han, G.; Han, N.; Yao, Z.; Wang, H.; et al. Nosocomial transmission of *Clostridium difficile* ribotype 027 in a Chinese hospital, 2012–2014, traced by whole genome sequencing. *BMC Genom.* **2016**, *17*, 405. [CrossRef] [PubMed]

69. Kim, H.; Lee, Y.; Moon, H.W.; Lim, C.S.; Lee, K.; Chong, Y. Emergence of *Clostridium difficile* ribotype 027 in Korea. *Korean J. Lab. Med.* **2011**, *31*, 191–196. [CrossRef] [PubMed]

70. Hung, Y.P.; Tsai, P.J.; Lee, Y.T.; Tang, H.J.; Lin, H.J.; Liu, H.C.; Lee, J.C.; Tsai, B.Y.; Hsueh, P.R.; Ko, W.C. Nationwide surveillance of ribotypes and antimicrobial susceptibilities of toxigenic *Clostridium difficile* isolates with an emphasis on reduced doxycycline and tigecycline susceptibilities among ribotype 078 lineage isolates in Taiwan. *Infect. Drug Resist.* **2018**, *11*, 1197–1203. [CrossRef]

71. Hung, Y.P.; Cia, C.T.; Tsai, B.Y.; Chen, P.C.; Lin, H.J.; Liu, H.C.; Lee, J.C.; Wu, Y.H.; Tsai, P.J.; Ko, W.C. The first case of severe *Clostridium difficile* ribotype 027 infection in Taiwan. *J. Infect.* **2015**, *70*, 98–101. [CrossRef]

72. Jin, H.; Ni, K.; Wei, L.; Shen, L.; Xu, H.; Kong, Q.; Ni, X. Identification of *Clostridium difficile* RT078 from patients and environmental surfaces in Zhejiang Province, China. *Infect. Control Hosp. Epidemiol.* **2016**, *37*, 745–746. [CrossRef]

73. Hung, Y.P.; Huang, I.H.; Lin, H.J.; Tsai, B.Y.; Liu, H.C.; Liu, H.C.; Lee, J.C.; Wu, Y.H.; Tsai, P.J.; Ko, W.C. Predominance of *Clostridium difficile* ribotypes 017 and 078 among toxigenic clinical isolates in southern Taiwan. *PLoS ONE* **2016**, *11*, e0166159. [CrossRef]

74. Seo, M.R.; Kim, J.; Lee, Y.; Lim, D.G.; Pai, H. Prevalence, genetic relatedness and antibiotic resistance of hospital-acquired *Clostridium difficile* PCR ribotype 018 strains. *Int. J. Antimicrob. Agents* **2018**, *51*, 762–767. [CrossRef] [PubMed]

75. Cheng, J.-W.; Xiao, M.; Kudinha, T.; Kong, F.; Xu, Z.-P.; Sun, L.-Y.; Zhang, L.; Fan, X.; Xie, X.-L.; Xu, Y.-C. Molecular epidemiology and antimicrobial susceptibility of *Clostridium difficile* isolates from a university teaching hospital in China. *Front. Microbiol.* **2016**, *7*, 1621. [CrossRef] [PubMed]

76. Chen, Y.B.; Gu, S.L.; Wei, Z.Q.; Shen, P.; Kong, H.S.; Yang, Q.; Li, L.J. Molecular epidemiology of *Clostridium difficile* in a tertiary hospital of China. *J. Med. Microbiol.* **2014**, *63*, 562–569. [CrossRef] [PubMed]

77. Wang, B.; Lv, Z.; Zhang, P.; Su, J. Molecular epidemiology and antimicrobial susceptibility of human *Clostridium difficile* isolates from a single institution in Northern China. *Medicine* **2018**, *97*, e11219. [CrossRef] [PubMed]

78. Tian, T.T.; Zhao, J.H.; Yang, J.; Qiang, C.X.; Li, Z.R.; Chen, J.; Xu, K.Y.; Ciu, Q.Q.; Li, R.X. Molecular characterization of *Clostridium difficile* isolates from human subjects and the environment. *PLoS ONE* **2016**, *11*, e0151964. [CrossRef] [PubMed]

79. Jin, D.; Luo, Y.; Huang, C.; Cai, J.; Ye, J.; Zheng, Y.; Wang, L.; Zhao, P.; Liu, A.; Fang, W.; et al. Molecular epidemiology of *Clostridium difficile* infection in hospitalized patients in Eastern China. *J. Clin. Microbiol.* **2017**, *55*, 801–810. [CrossRef] [PubMed]

80. Cheng, V.C.; Yam, W.C.; Lam, O.T.; Tsang, J.L.; Tse, E.Y.; Siu, G.K.; Chan, J.F.; Tse, H.; To, K.K.; Tai, J.W.; et al. *Clostridium difficile* isolates with increased sporulation: Emergence of PCR ribotype 002 in Hong Kong. *Eur. J. Clin. Microbiol. Infect. Dis.* **2011**, *30*, 1371–1381. [CrossRef]

81. Gao, Q.; Wu, S.; Huang, H.; Ni, Y.; Chen, Y.; Hu, Y.; Yu, Y. Toxin profiles, PCR ribotypes and resistance patterns of *Clostridium difficile*: A multicentre study in China, 2012–2013. *Int. J. Antimicrob. Agents* **2016**, *48*, 736–739. [CrossRef]

82. Gerding, D.N.; Meyer, T.; Lee, C.; Cohen, S.H.; Murthy, U.K.; Poirier, A.; Van Schooneveld, T.C.; Pardi, D.S.; Ramos, A.; Barron, M.A.; et al. Administration of spores of nontoxigenic *Clostridium difficile* strain M3 for prevention of recurrent *C. difficile* infection: A randomized clinical trial. *JAMA* **2015**, *313*, 1719–1727. [CrossRef]

83. Moura, I.; Spigaglia, P.; Barbanti, F.; Mastrantonio, P. Analysis of metronidazole susceptibility in different *Clostridium difficile* PCR ribotypes. *J. Antimicrob. Chemother.* **2013**, *68*, 362–365. [CrossRef]

84. Usui, M.; Nanbu, Y.; Oka, K.; Takahashi, M.; Inamatsu, T.; Asai, T.; Kamiya, S.; Tamura, Y. Genetic relatedness between Japanese and European isolates of *Clostridium difficile* originating from piglets and their risk associated with human health. *Front. Microbiol.* **2014**, *5*, 513. [CrossRef] [PubMed]

85. Kim, H.Y.; Cho, A.; Kim, J.W.; Kim, H.; Kim, B. High prevalence of *Clostridium difficile* PCR ribotype 078 in pigs in Korea. *Anaerobe* **2018**, *51*, 42–46. [CrossRef]

86. Wu, Y.C.; Lee, J.J.; Tsai, B.Y.; Liu, Y.F.; Chen, C.M.; Tien, N.; Tsai, P.J.; Chen, T.H. Potentially hypervirulent *Clostridium difficile* PCR ribotype 078 lineage isolates in pigs and possible implications for humans in Taiwan. *Int. J. Med. Microbiol.* **2016**, *306*, 115–122. [CrossRef] [PubMed]

87. Putsathit, P.; Ngamwongsatit, B.; Riley, T.V. Epidemiology and antimicrobial susceptibility of Clostridium difficile in piglets in Thailand. In Proceedings of the 6th International Clostridium difficile Symposium, Bled, Slovenia, 12–14 September 2018.

88. Hung, Y.P.; Lin, H.J.; Tsai, B.Y.; Liu, H.C.; Liu, H.C.; Lee, J.C.; Wu, Y.H.; Wilcox, M.H.; Fawley, W.N.; Hsueh, P.R.; et al. *Clostridium difficile* ribotype 126 in southern Taiwan: A cluster of three symptomatic cases. *Anaerobe* **2014**, *30*, 188–192. [CrossRef] [PubMed]

89. Baba, K.; Ishihara, K.; Ozawa, M.; Tamura, Y.; Asai, T. Isolation of meticillin-resistant *Staphylococcus aureus* (MRSA) from swine in Japan. *Int. J. Antimicrob. Agents* **2010**, *36*, 352–354. [CrossRef] [PubMed]

90. Spigaglia, P.; Drigo, I.; Barbanti, F.; Mastrantonio, P.; Bano, L.; Bacchin, C.; Puiatti, C.; Tonon, E.; Berto, G.; Agnoletti, F. Antibiotic resistance patterns and PCR-ribotyping of *Clostridium difficile* strains isolated from swine and dogs in Italy. *Anaerobe* **2015**, *31*, 42–46. [CrossRef]

91. Knight, D.R.; Putsathit, P.; Elliott, B.; Riley, T.V. Contamination of Australian newborn calf carcasses at slaughter with *Clostridium difficile*. *Clin. Microbiol. Infect.* **2016**, *22*, 266.e1–266.e7. [CrossRef]

92. Niwa, H.; Kato, H.; Hobo, S.; Kinoshita, Y.; Ueno, T.; Katayama, Y.; Hariu, K.; Oku, K.; Senoh, M.; Kuroda, T.; et al. Postoperative *Clostridium difficile* infection with PCR ribotype 078 strain identified at necropsy in five Thoroughbred racehorses. *Vet. Rec.* **2013**, *173*, 607. [CrossRef]

93. Niwa, H.; Sekizuka, T.; Kuroda, M.; Uchida, E.; Kinoshita, Y.; Katayama, Y.; Senoh, M.; Kato, H. Whole-genome analysis of Clostridioides difficile strains isolated from horses in Japan. In Proceedings of the 6th International Clostridium difficile Symposium, Bled, Slovenia, 12–14 September 2018.

94. Anderson, D.J.; Rojas, L.F.; Watson, S.; Knelson, L.P.; Pruitt, S.; Lewis, S.S.; Moehring, R.W.; Sickbert Bennett, E.E.; Weber, D.J.; Chen, L.F.; et al. Identification of novel risk factors for community-acquired *Clostridium difficile* infection using spatial statistics and geographic information system analyses. *PLoS ONE* **2017**, *12*, e0176285. [CrossRef]

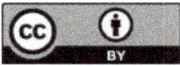

Tropical Medicine and Infectious Disease

MDPI

Opinion

The Importance of Wildlife Disease Monitoring as Part of Global Surveillance for Zoonotic Diseases: The Role of Australia

Rupert Woods [1,2,*], Andrea Reiss [1], Keren Cox-Witton [1], Tiggy Grillo [1] and Andrew Peters [3]

1   Wildlife Health Australia, Mosman, NSW 2088, Australia; areiss@wildlifehealthaustralia.com.au (A.R.);
     kcox-witton@wildlifehealthaustralia.com.au (K.C.-W.); tgrillo@wildlifehealthaustralia.com.au (T.G.)
2   World Organisation for Animal Health Working Group on Wildlife, 75017 Paris, France
3   School of Animal and Veterinary Sciences, E. H. Graham Centre for Agricultural Innovation,
     Charles Sturt University, Boorooma St., Wagga Wagga, New South Wales 2678, Australia;
     apeters@csu.edu.au
*   Correspondence: rwoods@wildlifehealthaustralia.com.au; Tel.: +61-043-875-5078

Received: 19 December 2018; Accepted: 31 January 2019; Published: 6 February 2019

Abstract: Australia has a comprehensive system of capabilities and functions to prepare, detect and respond to health security threats. Strong cooperative links and coordination mechanisms exist between the human (public health) and animal arms of the health system in Australia. Wildlife is included in this system. Recent reviews of both the animal and human health sectors have highlighted Australia's relative strengths in the detection and management of emerging zoonotic diseases. However, the risks to Australia posed by diseases with wildlife as part of their epidemiology will almost certainly become greater with changing land use and climate change and as societal attitudes bring wildlife, livestock and people into closer contact. These risks are not isolated to Australia but are global. A greater emphasis on wildlife disease surveillance to assist in the detection of emerging infectious diseases and integration of wildlife health into One Health policy will be critical in better preparing Australia and other countries in their efforts to recognize and manage the adverse impacts of zoonotic diseases on human health. Animal and human health practitioners are encouraged to consider wildlife in their day to day activities and to learn more about Australia's system and how they can become more involved by visiting www.wildlifeheathaustralia.com.au.

Keywords: Australia; emerging disease; international health regulations; Joint External Evaluation (JEE); One Health; Performance of Veterinary Services (PVS); surveillance; wildlife; zoonosis

---

1. Introduction

There is increasing recognition of the need to monitor as part of surveillance for emerging infectious diseases [1–4]. The majority of emerging infectious diseases are zoonoses with the predominant source shown to be wildlife [2,5]. Of specific concern is the impact and increase of wildlife-sourced zoonoses on human populations as globalisation, climate change and ecosystem alterations bring people and wildlife into closer contact. Importantly, many of the significant emerging infectious diseases in Australia have arisen in wildlife, and from within the country, rather than by overseas introductions, e.g., Hendra virus, Australian bat lyssavirus; see reviews [6,7]. For these reasons, Australia has implemented a general wildlife health surveillance system to enhance the early detection and characterization of microbial agents potentially involved with emerging diseases in free-ranging wildlife populations [6–8]. This paper briefly explains the governance for emerging zoonotic diseases and the roles played by non-human health professionals, especially those in the wildlife health sector in Australia. It concludes that though much good work has been done, there is an immediate need to improve integration of wildlife health into One Health policy as a critical step in better preparing Australia and other countries in their efforts to recognize and manage the adverse impacts of zoonotic diseases on human health.

2. Australia's Biosecurity System and Wildlife Health Systems

Australia is a federation of six states and two territories. The public and animal health (production animals, domestic animals and wildlife) systems are complex, with a number of participants across the three level of government (Australian, state or territory and local) and in different sectors (human, animal and environment) [9–11]. The nationalised, broad-ranging animal health biosecurity system and the wildlife health component have been previously described [6,12,13]. Australia's biosecurity system is complex, with activities carried out by Australian governments pre-border (offshore), border and post border (onshore) in collaboration with a large number of animal industry and other stakeholder groups, represented by a number of peak bodies. Under the Australian constitution, the Australian government is responsible for quarantine at the Australian border and also international animal health matters. State and territory governments are responsible for disease prevention, control and eradication within their boundaries. Preparedness plans and incident command structures adopted at both national and jurisdictional levels of government complement the system during emergency situations [11].

The framework ensures communication and cooperation between all levels of government and incorporates partnerships with animal industries and other stakeholders. An overarching National Animal Health Surveillance and Diagnostic Strategy Business Plan (Business Plan) guides investment in biosecurity priorities [14]. The wildlife component of the Business Plan focuses on nationally important and significant diseases of wildlife that may impact on Australia's animal industries, human health, biodiversity, trade and tourism ('wildlife diseases'). Emerging, exotic and zoonotic infectious diseases in addition to agriculturally significant diseases are emphasised.

Wildlife Health Australia (WHA) is a national body that works with Australian governments and stakeholders to improve preparedness, understanding and management of wildlife diseases. The current priority is the coordination of general surveillance and reporting of disease events in free-ranging wildlife. Over 30 surveillance partner agencies and organisations form the basis of Australia's general wildlife health surveillance system, which includes Australian, state and territory government agriculture and environment agencies, 10 zoos, eight private veterinary hospitals and seven universities around Australia. A number of targeted national programs are also in place, including a Bat Health Focus Group and the National Avian Influenza Wild Bird Surveillance Program [13]. Biosecurity, health and environment professionals are included in all of these programs, thus providing strong linkage across sectors. Recognition of the role of non-government stakeholders and the use of a partnership-type approach is a strength of the system.

A centralised, web-enabled national database of wildlife health information ('eWHIS') that is accessible across sectors by surveillance partners, both from within and outside of government, captures summary information on wildlife health and disease events submitted by surveillance partners in close to real time. About 40,000 wildlife cases are seen by WHA general surveillance partners each year [4] and one data category, 'Interesting or Unusual' wildlife cases, is designated to identify potential emerging infectious diseases. Within this category, between 200 and 300 'Interesting or Unusual' wildlife cases are reported in Australia each year.

3. Australia's Role in the Linkage and Coordination between Human and Animal Health Nationally and Internationally

Australia's capability across animal and human health has recently been evaluated by international assessors utilizing the World Health Organization's (WHO) Joint External Evaluation (JEE) against core capabilities and capacities under the International Health Regulations 2015, and the World Organisation for Animal Health's (OIE) Performance of Veterinary Services (PVS) Evaluation [9,11]. It was concluded that Australia has a comprehensive system of capabilities and functions for preparedness, detection and response to health security threats. Australia's system is strengthened through long-standing and stable cooperation links and coordination mechanisms that exist between the human and animal public health arms of the system [9]. The Australian Chief Veterinary Officer (ACVO) is Australia's delegate to the OIE (OIE Delegate). There is a need for the ACVO and Australia's state and territory Chief Veterinary Officers (CVOs) to maintain "line of sight" to the wildlife component of their animal health systems. Information provided by the wildlife surveillance system supports situation awareness and assessment of the risks posed by diseases of these animals. The ACVO coordinates Australia's OIE work and draws on other specialists in Australian Government departments and agencies, industry bodies and other sources of expertise. Strong linkage exists between the ACVO and CVOs, Australia's Chief Medical Officer and their respective departments [9]. Australia also has eight OIE Focal Points, focusing on specific animal-related topics such as wildlife, disease notification, communications and laboratories. These Focal Points support Australia's OIE Delegate and provide linkages with their counterparts in other countries through the OIE network [9].

The recent PVS evaluation also highlighted Australia's extraordinary commitment to biosecurity, serving the national interests by maintaining Australia's high animal health status. The very high level of biosecurity within Australian animal health is founded on strong partnership collaboration and formal business arrangements amongst jurisdictions and with the private sector, including primary producers, processors, suppliers of inputs and laboratories. The PVS evaluation, which also included wildlife, emphasised Australia's leadership role in the international veterinary community [11].

WHA supports the linkage and coordination between partners and across sectors by producing a regular electronic news digest that is distributed within Australia, to international members and regionally to OIE Wildlife Focal Points to share information on wildlife health and disease occurrences and issues of relevance to Australia and the region. Wildlife health surveillance data are summarised and publicly reported to the international community quarterly and yearly respectively via publications, namely Animal Health Surveillance Quarterly and Animal Health in Australia [15]. Summaries are also provided to OIE at six-monthly intervals, and WHA produces a six-month summary of Australian bat lyssavirus general surveillance data as "Bat Stats" [16]. Where possible, Australia's wildlife health data are also provided to open source databases (for example, the provision of sequence data generated by the Avian Influenza Wild Bird Surveillance Program to GenBank) and to help satisfy international reporting requirements (see [15,17]). Other relevant outputs coordinated by WHA include fact sheets and national biosecurity guidelines for wildlife health.

The processes in place for information capture, provision and reporting allow rapid and timely submission of wildlife health and disease information to the national system, assessment and notification to the relevant authorities.

4. Key Challenges and Opportunities Identified from the Australian Experience

Arguably the key challenge and opportunity emerging from Australia's experience in wildlife disease monitoring as part of surveillance for emerging infectious diseases is the difficulty in finding objective indicators of success [18]. Surveillance and response systems face considerable subjectivity if measurable outcomes, assessment and improvement of the efficacy and efficiency of wildlife disease preparedness remain lacking. Objectives for Australia's general wildlife health surveillance system are to:

- Improve Australia's ability to describe the occurrence and distribution of wildlife diseases.
- Allow early detection of unusual wildlife disease events including changes in the pattern of existing diseases and occurrence of emerging or exotic diseases.
- Provide basic data that is able to support more detailed *ad hoc* disease investigations.
- Provide data to support claims of freedom from specified diseases and answer queries from trading partners as requested.

- Identify and capture all sources of animal health information that would effectively contribute to Australia's overall understanding of its wildlife health.
- Remain highly cost effective and maximise the representativeness and coverage of the system.
- Improve and expand the capacity to collect information about feral animals, especially from non-government sources.

Seeking stakeholders' and users' input on how data and services provided by WHA improve their ability to identify and manage wildlife disease risk and preparedness is a good example of the pragmatic approach to measure success that is currently used. Effective detection and eradication of emerging infectious diseases in wildlife requires the collection of objective evidence to demonstrate the robustness of wildlife disease monitoring systems. This information, in turn, will guide adequate deployment of resources and implementation of system improvements. We are not aware of any examples of emerging infectious diseases of Australian native wildlife that have been eradicated or locally eliminated by Australian state or territory governments. A discussion of tools and tactics is beyond the scope of this opinion piece but includes options routinely deployed in production, invasive and feral animal response. Though local elimination and or proof of eradication appear to be conceptually simple measures of success, a common indicator used in human and animal health economics, economic loss averted (ELA), could also be deployed. Despite some of the challenges, the use of ELA would not only allow a greater understanding of the benefit cost of the system, but also allow comparisons to be made with other national animal and human health risk mitigation programs.

Wildlife disease surveillance faces other recognised challenges. There is incomplete knowledge of wildlife population demographics and distributions, as well as legitimate questions of surveillance sensitivity and potential biases in results. Australia uses a pragmatic approach, focusing on the development of a good general surveillance system, rapid reporting, as well as the identification and investigation of clusters of wildlife deaths or morbidity. The supporting architecture for the wildlife health surveillance system is based on Australia's livestock biosecurity framework and has historically focussed on the capture and provision of information to support trade and market access. Recognising that a general surveillance system to support one sector also supports others, a greater focus on zoonotic diseases and diseases which may impact wildlife populations and biodiversity and their inclusion in general surveillance activities would significantly strengthen the Australian system. The recent work of Craik, Palmer and Sheldrake [10] concluded that there was an immediate need to further invest in environmental biosecurity and bring it more fully into mainstream biosecurity activities in Australia. The inclusion of the environmental sector in arrangements targeting wildlife health and diseases in Australia would significantly improve the ability to detect new and emerging diseases with the potential to impact upon animal and or human health. The recent appointment of a Chief Environmental Biosecurity Officer for Australia (ACEBO) is a significant development that offers opportunities in improving the coordination and linkage between environment, health and agriculture.

More broadly, there remains significant opportunity for improvement of the position of wildlife within Australia's wider biosecurity arrangements. There are challenges, however, with maintaining a high operational functionality in Australia's complex system. The JEE concluded that despite outstanding progress in developing and implementing steps to ensure a collaborative approach between the human and animal health sectors, opportunities remain for the development of greater coordination of activities [9]. Given the risks posed by anthropogenic changes that have the potential to spark disease outbreaks in wildlife populations and the potential emergence of zoonotic diseases, each of the observations proposed by the JEE could be enhanced by the further consideration and inclusion of wildlife and environmental health:

- Development of an all-hazards health protection framework. The national framework for communicable disease control could be further developed with an increased emphasis on the risks posed by anthropogenic changes to the environment, which are linked to disease emergence in wildlife, changes in relative distribution and composition of infectious agents and species affected.

- Public and animal health workforce issues. Some specific competencies were recognized for which there is a limited workforce and future replacement may be at risk. For wildlife, this includes disease ecologists and disease and wildlife emergency response managers. Australia's PVS evaluation noted that in several jurisdictions staff levels are seen to be severely inadequate [11]. Increased investment in on-the-ground veterinary officer deployment for investigation and surveillance activities is required. Only some of Australia's environmental agencies include veterinarians and a placement within each of these agencies would also facilitate communication and linkage with counterparts in agriculture and public health agencies.
- The use of genomic data in disease surveillance, which could be better harnessed for pathogen discovery, surveillance work and elucidating the epidemiology at population interfaces, for example, at the wildlife–human and wildlife–livestock interfaces. A sequence data management and interpretation framework bridging bio-informatics and evolutionary microbiology (phylogenetics, phylogeography) is of critical importance in comprehensively holistic programs, particularly to provide an adequate ecological and evolutionary interpretation of the relationships between agents discovered in wildlife and zoonotic agents affecting human populations. All of this has the ultimate purpose of tracing the potential origins of zoonotic diseases, unveiling mechanisms as to how wildlife-associated agents may break cross species transmission barriers (host shifts) or simply quantifying and qualifying transient cross-species spillover infections. The European COMPARE project is an example of an effective approach to tackling emerging infectious diseases, ranging from risk assessment, sampling frames and surveillance, application of new generation sequencing, and data flow into databases, to the development of harmonized approaches across human, livestock and wildlife populations [19].
- Joint training and emergency animal disease response exercises across Australian Government agencies, relevant state and territory government agencies, and wildlife stakeholders, along with strategic risk assessment of current preparedness activities and arrangements for wildlife, would help to identify areas requiring improvement.
- Wildlife monitoring also presents an opportunity to assist with linkage across sectors in the areas of surveillance, preparedness and investigation. However, simpler management structures are required and the use of WHA, a public-private partnership built on One Health principles, to assist as a "trusted broker" represents a potential opportunity for the system that needs to be further developed.
- Information technology and mapping systems between Australian jurisdictions are not yet fully compatible [11]. Linkage of jurisdictional information systems to the eWHIS would remove redundancy, improve efficiency and allow analysis at a whole of country scale.

Following the completion of a JEE, the WHO recommends that countries develop a National Action Plan for Health Security (NAPHS) to address the recommendations in the JEE Mission Report. In keeping with the JEE ideology, the NAPHS is developed collaboratively across multiples sectors, with the aim of prioritising the implementation of recommendations to improve compliance with international health regulations and national health security. Specific recommendations for zoonotic diseases in Australia's NAPHS are:

- "Introduce a formal process through committee structures between human health and animal health to regularly review a joint list of priority zoonotic diseases. Consider designating zoonotic diseases of public health importance in Australia as nationally notifiable in animals.
- Establish a dedicated multisectoral national zoonosis committee or ensure reciprocal animal and human sector representation on their respective national zoonotic disease-related committees to enhance communications, bridge knowledge gaps and strengthen collaborative responses.
- Consider standardising/aligning laboratory case definitions and typing between human and animal health sectors to enhance data comparison of their surveillance systems [20]".

In addressing these recommendations, it is important for Australia that emerging infectious diseases and zoonoses of wildlife be included.

5. Conclusions

The risks to Australia posed by wildlife diseases will almost certainly become greater with anthropogenic changes such as a climate change, changes in land use, as well as societal attitudes that bring wildlife, livestock and people into closer contact [6]. The challenges of emerging infectious diseases from wildlife is, however, a global issue. A greater emphasis on wildlife disease surveillance to assist in the detection of emerging infectious diseases and integration of wildlife and environmental health into One Health policy will be critical in better preparing Australia and other countries in their efforts to recognize and manage the adverse impacts of zoonotic diseases on human health. Animal and human health professionals, including those in the community, are reminded of Australia's system of arrangements for wildlife health and are encouraged to consider wildlife health in their practices. More information on Australia's system and how they can become involved and contribute to improving the integration of wildlife health into their practice and communicate within an evolving network of partners is available at www.wildlifehealthaustralia.com.au.

Author Contributions: R.W. led the work which was co-authored by A.R., K.C.-W., T.G. and A.P.

Funding: The work of WHA is funded under a cost shared agreement between all Australian governments with oversight provided by Australia's National Biosecurity Committee.

Acknowledgments: Comments from Andrew Breed, Jenny Firman, Rachel Iglesias, Gary Lum, Mark Schipp, members of WHA's management committee and three anonymous reviewers significantly improved the manuscript.

Conflicts of Interest: Woods, Cox-Witton, Grillo and Reiss assist Australian governments and partners in administering Australia's wildlife health surveillance system and work for the national coordinating body, WHA.

References

1. Kruse, H.; Kirkemo, A.M.; Handeland, K. Wildlife as source of zoonotic infections. *Emerg. Infect. Dis.* **2004**, *10*, 2067–2072. [CrossRef] [PubMed]
2. Jones, K.E.; Patel, N.G.; Levy, M.A.; Storeygard, A.; Balk, D.; Gittleman, J.L.; Daszak, P. Global trends in emerging infectious diseases. *Nature* **2008**, *451*, 990–993. [CrossRef] [PubMed]
3. Sleeman, J.; Brand, C.; Wright, S. Strategies for wildlife disease surveillance. In *New Directions in Conservation Medicine*; Aguirre, A., Ostfeld, R., Daszak, P., Eds.; Oxford University Press: New York, NY, USA, 2012; pp. 539–551.
4. Cox-Witton, K.; Reiss, A.; Woods, R.; Grillo, V.; Baker, R.T.; Blyde, D.J.; Boardman, W.; Cutter, S.; Lacasse, C.; McCracken, H.; et al. Emerging infectious diseases in free-ranging wildlife–Australian zoo based wildlife hospitals contribute to national surveillance. *PLoS ONE* **2014**, *9*, e95127. [CrossRef] [PubMed]
5. McFarlane, R.; Sleigh, A.; McMichael, T. Synanthropy of wild mammals as a determinant of emerging infectious diseases in the Asian-Australasian region. *Ecohealth* **2012**, *9*, 24–35. [CrossRef] [PubMed]
6. Woods, R.; Grillo, T. Wildlife health in Australia. In *Medicine of Australian Mammals—CVT*; Vogelnest, L., Portas, T., Eds.; CSIRO: Sydney, Australia, 2019.
7. Reiss, A. Emerging infectious diseases. In *Medicine of Australian Mammals—CVT*; Vogelnest, L., Portas, T., Eds.; CSIRO: Sydney, Australia, 2019.
8. Woods, R.; Bunn, C. Wildlife health surveillance in Australia. *Microbiol. Aust.* **2005**, *26*, 56–58.
9. World Health Organization. *Joint External Evaluation of IHR Core Capacities of Australia: Mission Report, 24 November–1 December 2017*; World Health Organization: Geneva, Switzerland, 2018.
10. Craik, W.; Palmer, D.; Sheldrake, R. *Priorities for Australia's Biosecurity System: An Independent Review of the Capacity of the National Biosecurity System and Its Underpinning Intergovernmental Agreement*; Department of Agriculture and Water Resources: Canberra, Australia, 2017.
11. Schneider, H.; Batho, H.; Stermshorn, B.; Thiermann, A. *PVS Evaluation Report, Australia*; World Organisation for Animal Health: Paris, France, November, 2015.
12. Animal Health Australia. *Animal Health in Australia 2016*; Animal Health Australia: Canberra, Australia, 2017.

13. Wildlife Health Australia. National Wildlife Health Information System. Available online: https://www.wildlifehealthaustralia.com.au/ProgramsProjects/eWHISWildlifeHealthInformationSystem.aspx (accessed on 22 November 2018).

14. Department of Agriculture and Water Resources. *National Animal Health Surveillance and Diagnostics Business Plan 2016–2019*; Department of Agriculture and Water Resources: Canberra, Australia, 2016.

15. Animal Health Australia. *Animal Health in Australia 2017*; Animal Health Australia: Canberra, Australia, 2018.

16. WHA Bat Health Focus Group. *ABLV Bat Stats*; WHA Bat Health Focus Group: Sydney, Australia, 2018.

17. Grillo, T.; Arzey, K.E.; Hansbro, P.M.; Hurt, A.C.; Warner, S.; Bergfeld, J.; Burgess, G.W.; Cookson, B.; Dickason, C.J.; Ferenczi, M.; et al. Avian influenza in Australia: A summary of 5 years of wild bird surveillance. *Aust. Vet. J.* **2015**, *93*, 387–393. [CrossRef] [PubMed]

18. Nguyen, N.T.; Duff, J.P.; Gavier-Widén, D.; Grillo, T.; He, H.; Lee, H.; Ratanakorn, P.; Rijks, J.M.; Ryser-Degiorgis, M.-P.; Sleeman, J.M. *Report of the Workshop on Evidence-Based Design of National Wildlife Health Programs*; US Department of the Interior US Geological Survey: Reston, VA, USA, 2017.

19. Compare. About Compare. Available online: https://www.compare-europe.eu/about (accessed on 19 December 2018).

20. Department of Health. *Australia's National Action Plan for Health Security 2019–2023*; Department of Health: Canberra, Australia, 2018.

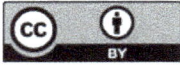

Tropical Medicine and
Infectious Disease

MDPI

Article

Insights into Australian Bat Lyssavirus in Insectivorous Bats of Western Australia

Diana Prada [1,*], Victoria Boyd [2], Michelle Baker [2], Bethany Jackson [1,†] and Mark O'Dea [1,†]

1   School of Veterinary Medicine, Murdoch University, Perth, WA 6150, Australia;
    b.jackson@murdoch.edu.au (B.J.); m.odea@murdoch.edu.au (M.O.)
2   Australian Animal Health Laboratory, CSIRO, Geelong, VIC 3220, Australia; vicky.boyd@csiro.au (V.B.);
    michelle.baker@csiro.au (M.B.)
*   Correspondence: 32589004@student.murdoch.edu.au; Tel.: +61-893607418
†   These authors contributed equally.

Received: 21 February 2019; Accepted: 7 March 2019; Published: 11 March 2019

Abstract: Australian bat lyssavirus (ABLV) is a known causative agent of neurological disease in bats, humans and horses. It has been isolated from four species of pteropid bats and a single microbat species (*Saccolaimus flaviventris*). To date, ABLV surveillance has primarily been passive, with active surveillance concentrating on eastern and northern Australian bat populations. As a result, there is scant regional ABLV information for large areas of the country. To better inform the local public health risks associated with human-bat interactions, this study describes the lyssavirus prevalence in microbat communities in the South West Botanical Province of Western Australia. We used targeted real-time PCR assays to detect viral RNA shedding in 839 oral swabs representing 12 species of microbats, which were sampled over two consecutive summers spanning 2016–2018. Additionally, we tested 649 serum samples via Luminex® assay for reactivity to lyssavirus antigens. Active lyssavirus infection was not detected in any of the samples. Lyssavirus antibodies were detected in 19 individuals across six species, with a crude prevalence of 2.9% (95% CI: 1.8–4.5%) over the two years. In addition, we present the first records of lyssavirus exposure in two *Nyctophilus* species, and *Falsistrellus mackenziei*.

Keywords: Australian bat lyssavirus; microbats; Western Australia; serology; Luminex; real-time PCR

1. Introduction

Australian bat lyssavirus (ABLV) is one of the 16 classified species of lyssaviruses within the family *Rhabdoviridae* [1]. It was first discovered in Australia in 1996 [2] and early studies distinguished two variants, the pteropid variant carried by all four species of flying fox within continental Australia [3], and the insectivorous variant detected only in the yellow-bellied sheath-tailed bat (*Saccolaimus flaviventris*) [4]. Although there is evidence of ABLV exposure in 11 genera within four microbat families [5], additional reservoir species have yet to be identified.

Both ABLV strains are associated with clinical disease in the host species [2,4]. Although spillover events are extremely rare, they have resulted in fatal neurological disease in humans and horses [6–8], making ABLV an agent of significant public health concern. Current public health policy recommends a prophylactic rabies vaccination for bat handlers, with the administration of post-exposure treatment including vaccination and rabies immunoglobulin based on vaccination history and individual immune status [9]. However, the perceived risk from exposure to microbats is potentially limited by the relative lack of media exposure these species receive compared to the larger pteropids, coupled with only a single documented microbat to human transmission of ABLV to date.

Since the discovery of ABLV, surveillance has predominantly relied on passive sampling regimes, with a single published study based on active sampling in the east and north of the country [10].

Trop. Med. Infect. Dis. **2019**, *4*, 46

Results suggest ABLV circulates at a low prevalence (<1%) in healthy wild bat populations [5]. However, the prevalence (and therefore risk) escalates to 5%–10% where bats are injured, sick or orphaned. These are precisely the conditions which are considered to drive human exposure through rescue and rehabilitation attempts, or the protection of property, pets or children [11–13]. Interestingly, the public health research on ABLV and human-bat interactions to date does not report on community knowledge or risk perceptions of microbats versus pteropid species, generally referring to 'bats' as a broad group [11–15]. Therefore, whilst basic knowledge of ABLV in bats appears to be high in some regions [11], public awareness of the specific risks and recommended post-exposure behaviours with respect to microbats warrants further research.

In Western Australia, ABLV surveillance has also been sporadic and passive, with the only targeted study focusing on the far northern part of the state and concentrating mainly on the pteropid bats in the region [5], with sample collection occurring some 15 years ago. Active surveillance of microbats has likely been hindered by the additional time and resource demands of sampling non-cave roosting species typical of the region [16]. Therefore, there is limited current information on the ABLV status of Western Australian microbat species and the disease status is assumed by the extrapolation of information from bat populations in the eastern states. Additionally, there is no local data of ABLV status in the south west of Western Australia, an area with arguably increased human-bat interaction due to the higher population density.

In order to better inform the regional risks associated with human-bat interactions, this study aimed to establish the lyssavirus status of insectivorous bats in the South-West Botanical Province of WA over a period of two years. We used an ABLV specific and a pan-lyssavirus reverse transcription real-time PCR (RRT-PCR) assay to screen oral swabs from 12 species of microbats. Additionally, we used a bead-based Luminex® assay on serum samples to determine previous lyssavirus exposure.

2. Materials and Methods

All sampling was approved by the Department of Parks and Wildlife of Western Australia, permits 08-001359-1, and CE005517. Capture, handling and sampling procedures were approved by the Murdoch University Animal Ethics Committee (R2882/16).

Harp traps and mist nets were used to capture bats at different locations of the South-West Botanical Province (SWBP), an Australian global biodiversity hotspot. The province covers approximately 44 million hectares and comprises nine bioregions [17]. Remnant natural cover in the east and west of the region is separated by the extensive monoculture known as the Western Australian wheatbelt, which acts as a major dispersion barrier for many native species.

Sampling took place over two summers between 2016 and 2018, with sites in the east and west boundaries of the wheatbelt. The northeastern sites were within the semi-arid Avon bioregion which was predominantly sampled during the first season (2016–2017). The southwestern sites were distributed across five bioregions, the Esperance Plains, Geraldton Sandplains, Jarrah Forest, Swan Coastal Plain, and Warren (Figure 1), which were mainly sampled during the second year of the study (2017–2018). Therefore, most sampling sites were visited only once over the two years, except for locations in the Avon bioregion which were sampled during both summers.

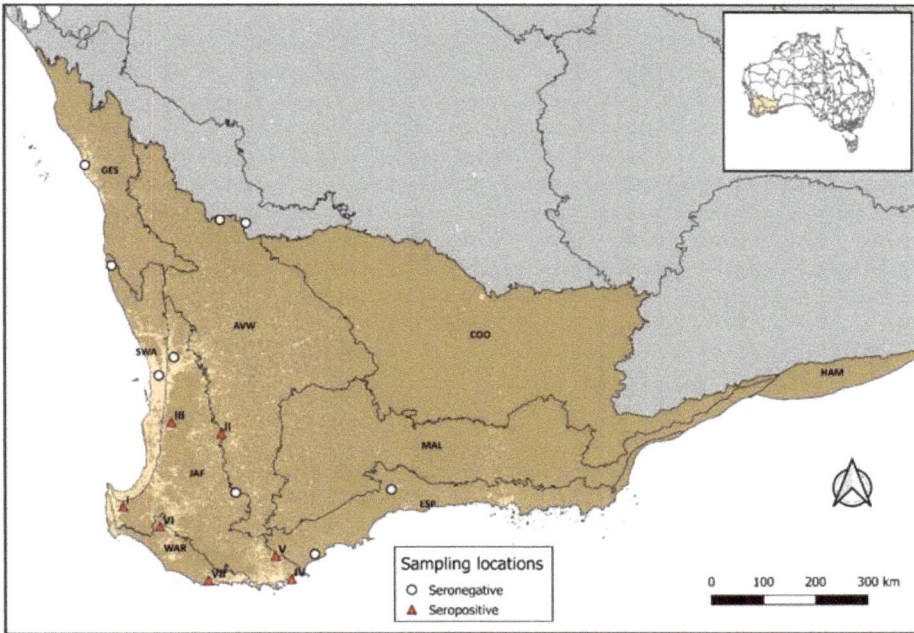

Figure 1. The South West Botanical province (SWBP) highlighted in brown. Sampling sites are shown and sites where seropositive individuals were identified are labelled I-VII. Presence (light areas) and absence (dark areas) of human populations are shown. The SWBP encompasses nine bioregions, Avon Wheatbelt (AVW), Coolgardie (COO), Esperance Plains (ESP), Geraldton Sandplains (GES), Hampton (HAM), Jarrah Forest (JAF), Mallee (MAL), Swan Coastal Plain (SWA), and Warren (WAR).

Prior to undertaking trapping, all personnel involved in handling bats underwent a complete rabies vaccination schedule. Biosecurity and biosafety protocols during handling and sampling included the use of protective gloves while manipulating bats out of traps and nets. During sample collection, double gloves were worn while restraining the animal (nitrile gloves over protective gloves), with the nitrile gloves changed between each bat. All surfaces and non-disposable equipment (e.g., calipers) were disinfected with a 10% solution of F10 (Health and Hygiene, South Africa) between each bat. Additionally, single calico bags were used for each individual and soaked in F10 before being re-used.

Following capture, bats were taxonomically identified, and a single oral swab (FLOQSwab, Copan, Brescia, Italy) was collected per individual and stored in RNAlater® (Ambion, Life Technologies, Carlsbad, CA, USA). Additionally, 10 μL of blood was taken from the brachial vein and diluted 1:10 in phosphate buffered saline (PBS).

Oral swabs were vortexed and 50 μL of the supernatant used as starting material for all extractions using a Magmax viral RNA extraction kit (Ambion, Applied Biosystems, Vilnius, Lithuania) following the manufacturer's instructions. The detection of lyssavirus RNA was performed using an Australian bat lyssavirus RRT-PCR specific for the insectivorous variant of the virus [18], and a pan-lyssavirus RRT-PCR assay [19]. Inactivated insectivorous ABLV RNA provided by the CSIRO Australian Animal Health Laboratory (AAHL, Victoria, Australia) was used as a positive control. Assays were performed on a QuantStudio 6 Flex platform (Life Technologies, Singapore). Nucleic acid extraction verification and lack of inhibitors were assessed using an endogenous 18S rRNA PCR assay (Life Technologies, Pleasanton, CA, USA).

Sera were tested for reactivity to lyssavirus antigens [20] in an indirect binding Luminex®
assay [21], at a final working dilution of 1:50 at CSIRO AAHL. As a pilot study, samples collected
during the first season were pooled one in three (*n* = 246) or one in four (*n* = 24). All samples collected
during the second season were tested individually (*n* = 391). Median Fluorescence Intensity (MFI)
was read using a Bio-Plex instrument (Bio-Rad Laboratories, Hercules, CA, USA). Due to the lack
of known positive and known negative bat sera from the species captured in this study to validate
the assay, the MFI threshold to differentiate positive and negative samples was set at 1000 MFI as
per CSIRO protocols. Previous studies published by the Australian Animal Health Laboratory and
elsewhere using the same Bio-Plex platform have used a threshold of at least three times the mean
MFI of negative sera from other bat species with values below 250 MFI considered negative [22–25].
The same principle was used here to establish a threshold based on an MFI of 250 corresponding to a
negative sample with sample MFIs above 1000 considered positive.

Prevalence estimates and 95% confidence intervals were calculated using the Wilson's Method [26]
as implemented in the R package *epitools* [27].

3. Results

In total, 839 oral swabs and 661 blood samples were collected. Twelve samples did not provide
a valid Luminex® assay result and were removed from the analysis. Therefore, the final serological
dataset comprised 649 samples encompassing 12 bat species (Table 1). Captured species composition
varied at each location (Figure 2) and in general *Chalinolobus gouldii* and *Vespadelus regulus* had the
greatest representation in the swab and sera data sets (Table 1). A total of 270 serum samples were
collected in the first year and 379 during the second year.

Table 1. Seroprevalence of Australian Bat Lyssavirus in 12 species of microbats of the South West
Botanical Province of Western Australia. The total number of samples tested and positives () are shown.

Family	Species	Swabs	Sera	Seroprevalence [1]
Vespertilionidae	*Chalinolobus gouldii*	287(0)	262(2)	0.7 (0.2–2.7)
	Chalinolobus morio	105(0)	64(3)	4.6 (1.6–12.8)
	Falsistrellus mackenziei	14(0)	7(1)	NC [2]
	Nyctophilus geoffroyi	69(0)	48(0)	
	Nyctophilus gouldi	78(0)	66(3)	4.5 (1.5–12.5)
	Nyctophilus major	12(0)	5(1)	NC [2]
	Nyctophilus sp [3]	6(0)	5(0)	
	Scotorepens balstoni	13(0)	8(0)	
	Vespadelus baverstocki	6(0)	5(0)	
	Vespadelus finlaysoni	1(0)	0	
	Vespadelus regulus	227(0)	164(9)	5.5 (2.9–10.1)
	Vespadelus sp [3]	2(0)	1(0)	
Molossidae	*Austronomus australis*	13(0)	11(0)	
	Ozimops sp	6(0)	3(0)	

[1] Prevalence (%) and 95% confidence intervals (CI). [2] Prevalence estimates not calculated (NC) due to small sample
size. [3] These individuals were not confidently identified to species level, however will belong to either of the listed
Nyctophilus or *Vespadelus* species, and therefore do not count towards the total number of species sampled.

Neither the ABLV specific or the pan-lyssavirus RRT-PCR reactions yielded a positive result.
No inhibition was detected in any of the samples and positive and negative controls were valid.

Serological reactivity to lyssavirus antigens was detected in 19 samples (Table 1, Table S1) resulting
in an overall antibody prevalence of 2.9% (95% CI: 1.8–4.5%). Seropositive samples encompassed six
species, *V. regulus* had the highest prevalence at 5.5% (95% CI: 2.9–10.1%), followed by *C. morio* (4.6%,
95% CI: 1.6–12.8), *Nyctophilus gouldi* (4.5%, 95% CI: 1.5–12.5) and *C. gouldii* (0.7%, 95% CI: 0.2–2.7%).
Additionally, reactivity was also detected in a single *Falsistrellus mackenziei*, and an *N. major*. Due to
their small sample sizes, prevalence values were not estimated for these two species (Table 1).

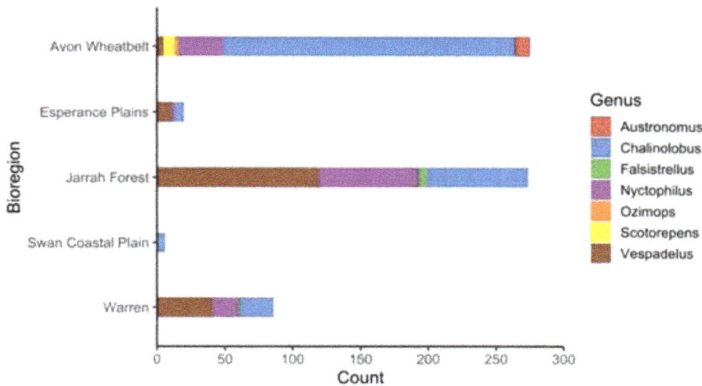

Figure 2. Number of blood samples taken by genera and bioregion. Note, no blood samples were obtained from bats in the Geraldton Sandplains bioregion.

Despite a large number of individuals being sampled during the first year (n = 270), none reacted on the lyssavirus serological assay, thus all seropositive bats were captured during the second year of the study, and south of the wheatbelt. Consequently, annual seroprevalence significantly increased from 0% in the first year to 5% (95% CI: 3.2–7.7%) in the second year (p = < 0.0001). It should be noted that the majority (78%) of captures in the first year and north of the wheatbelt were dominated by a single species, *C. gouldii*.

Seropositive individuals were captured at seven sites which were dominated by natural jarrah (*Eucalyptus marginata)* and marri (*Corymbia calophylla*) forests, and on one occasion on agricultural land transitioning to wandoo (*E. wandoo*) woodlands (Table 2). Seropositive *V. regulus* were sampled at five different locations, seropositive *N. gouldii*, and *C. morio* were captured at three and two locations, respectively, and the remaining two species were all captured at a single site. When examining the data by number of seropositive samples per location, three different species were captured at three locations, and the remaining four locations were represented by a single seropositive species.

Table 2. Distribution of seropositive individuals per bioregion and trapping location. Number of positives () per species.

Bioregion	Location	Species
Jarrah Forest	I	*Vespadelus regulus* (1)
	II	*Chalinolobus gouldii* (2)
	III	*Vespadelus regulus* (2)
		Nyctophilus major (1)
		Falsistrellus mackenziei (1)
	IV	*Nyctophilus gouldi* (1)
	V	*Vespadelus regulus* (1)
Warren	VI	*Chalinolobus morio* (2)
		Nyctophilus gouldi (1)
		Vespadelus regulus (1)
	VII	*Chalinolobus morio* (1)
		Nyctophilus gouldi (1)
		Vespadelus regulus (4)

4. Discussion

Here we report the first comprehensive study investigating the lyssavirus status of apparently healthy populations of insectivorous bats in the South West Botanical Province of WA. Significantly, this is the first active surveillance to take place in the SWBP and therefore constitutes an update to the existing limited lyssavirus data on wild microbat populations [10]. We did not detect any current ABLV infection or the presence of any other lyssavirus species circulating within the sampled populations, despite the large sample size (*n* = 839). The suitability of oral swabs for lyssavirus detection has previously been demonstrated in clinical studies [18,28–30], and in active lyssavirus surveillance efforts [31,32]. Nonetheless, diagnostic sensitivity in a field surveillance setting for the detection of ABLV may be limited by the combination of intermittent shedding [33], and a small window of infection [32,34] of an already low prevalence virus.

Serological results indicated previous lyssavirus exposure in 19 individuals, resulting in an overall seroprevalence of 2.9% in the study population. This result is congruent with previous sero-response estimates of wild Australian bat populations [5], albeit using a different serological assay. Antibody reactivity was detected in six Vespertilionidae species, *C. gouldii, C. morio, V. regulus, F. mackenziei, N. gouldi,* and *N. major*. The presence of lyssavirus antibodies has previously been documented for the *Chalinolobus* and *Vespadelus* genera [5], and the results here constitute the first published report of lyssavirus exposure in *Nyctophilus spp.* and *F. mackenziei*, an endemic species of the jarrah forests of the South West. It was not possible to carry out further confirmatory testing on seropositive individuals, as the volume of blood ethically permissible to be drawn from microbats was fully used in the Luminex® assay.

Seroprevalence values per species varied between 0.7% and 5.5%, with the highest values observed in *V. regulus* (5.5%), *C. morio* (4.6%) and *N. gouldi* (4.5%). Despite the existence of previously published seroprevalence figures for some Australian Vespertilionidae species [5], it is not appropriate to make direct comparisons due to previous results grouping different species by genera and being based on an alternative serological assay. Even though seropositivity for ABLV has previously been reported in *Austronomus australis* [5], we did not detect any antibody response in this species, possibly due to the small sample size (*n* = 11).

All seropositive individuals originated from seven locations within the Jarrah and Warren bioregions and none from the Avon bioregion, which is isolated by the Australian wheatbelt. It is unclear whether this partitioning of the data represents a geographical, temporal or a species association given these risk factors are confounded in the study population. However, temporal shedding may explain the 0% prevalence in the Avon bioregion despite the large sample size (*n* = 226), as this region was predominantly sampled in the first year and all the seropositive individuals occurred in the second year of the study. This hypothesis is supported by longitudinal studies elsewhere showing that inter-annual variation of seroprevalence estimates is common in wild bat populations [28,32]. Further, long term active surveillance in *Myotis myotis* has provided important insights into the infection dynamics of lyssavirus at a temporal and geographical scale [32], highlighting how similar studies would contribute to better understanding of ABLV dynamics within Australian microbat populations. It is possible that a failure to detect seropositive samples during the first year could also have been the result of decreased assay sensitivity triggered by sample pooling. However, titration studies using pools of *Pteropus alecto* sera by CSIRO AAHL have not demonstrated a loss of assay sensitivity at the pooling levels used in this study.

The detection of ABLV seropositivity in the SWBP, particularly the southern parts of the region, further supports the existence of additional lyssavirus reservoirs, as the distribution of *Pteropus spp.* and *Saccolaimus flaviventris* does not extend to the SWBP. This suggests that any hypothetical reservoir may be a member of the families Vespertilionidae or Molossidae, with serology results indicating Vespertilionidae may be a reservoir genus in the Southwest of WA. Importantly, seropositive individuals of six separate species came from a variety of areas in the south west in relatively close proximity to towns and recreational areas (<20 km).

The results from this study suggest that active infections in wild microbat populations may be even lower than previously thought. Despite this, the evidence of circulating ABLV in the region validates current recommendations for post-exposure treatment of people with bat bites and scratches, including those from microbats. We recommend public health research akin to that conducted in the eastern states [11–15] in order to evaluate knowledge, attitudes and perceptions of ABLV risks in the south west of WA specifically for microbat species. This information should be used to guide future public health campaigns in the region.

Supplementary Materials: The following are available online at http://www.mdpi.com/2414-6366/4/1/46/s1, Table S1 Median Fluoresce Intensity values for all sera tested.

Author Contributions: M.O., B.J. and D.P. designed the study and collected the data; V.B. and M.B. carried out all the serology laboratory work; D.P. performed all the molecular laboratory work and analysed the data from the molecular and serology datasets; D.P. drafted the manuscript; M.O. and B.J. reviewed and edited the manuscript; M.O. and B.J. supervised the research.

Funding: This research was funded by the Murdoch University Small Grants Scheme, Gunduwa Regional Conservation Association, the Holsworth Wildlife Research Endowment, The Australian Wildlife Society University Grants (2016) and the Alistair Bursary (2017).

Acknowledgments: We would like to acknowledge all the volunteers involved in the data collection. This project would not have been possible without their help and good disposition in the field. We would also like to thank Robert Bullen, Nicholas Dunlop, Terry Reardon, Andrew Grigg and Cameron Richardson from Alcoa, and members of the Department of Biodiversity, Conservation and Attractions in particular Sarah Comber, Janine Liddelow, and Peter Lacey for their assistance in identifying adequate bat trapping sites, which was fundamental to this project. We also thank the private landowners who provided access to their properties, as well as John and Lisa Lawson from the Lions Dryandra Village for facilitating our stay there. We would also like to thank the Australian Wildlife Conservancy and Bush Heritage Australia for supporting this project.

Conflicts of Interest: The authors declare no conflict of interest. The funders had no role in the design of the study; in the collection, analyses, or interpretation of data; in the writing of the manuscript, or in the decision to publish the results.

References

1. International Committee on Taxonomy of Viruses. Available online: https://talk.ictvonline.org/taxonomy/ (accessed on 14 February 2019).
2. Fraser, G.C.; Hooper, P.T.; Lunt, R.A.; Gould, A.R.; Gleeson, L.J.; Hyatt, A.D.; Russell, G.M.; Kattenbelt, J.A. Encephalitis Caused by a Lyssavirus in Fruit Bats in Australia. *Emerg. Infect. Dis.* **1996**, *2*, 327–331. [CrossRef] [PubMed]
3. Gould, A.R.; Hyatt, A.D.; Lunt, R.; Kattenbelt, J.A.; Hengstberger, S.; Blacksell, S. Characterisation of a novel lyssavirus isolated from Pteropid bats in Australia. *Virus Res.* **1998**, *54*, 165–187. [CrossRef]
4. Gould, A.R.; Kattenbelt, J.A.; Gumley, S.G.; Lunt, R.A. Characterisation of an Australian bat lyssavirus variant isolated from an insectivorous bat. *Virus Res.* **2002**, *89*, 1–28. [CrossRef]
5. Field, H.E. Evidence of Australian bat lyssavirus infection in diverse Australian bat taxa. *Zoonoses Public Health* **2018**, *65*, 742–748. [CrossRef] [PubMed]
6. Francis, J.R.; Nourse, C.; Vaska, V.L.; Calvert, S.; Northill, J.A.; McCall, B.; Mattke, A.C. Australian Bat Lyssavirus in a child: The first reported case. *Pediatrics* **2014**, *133*, e1063–e1067. [CrossRef] [PubMed]
7. Shinwari, M.W.; Annand, E.J.; Driver, L.; Warrilow, D.; Harrower, B.; Allcock, R.J.N.; Pukallus, D.; Harper, J.; Bingham, J.; Kung, N.; et al. Australian bat lyssavirus infection in two horses. *Vet. Microbiol.* **2014**, *173*, 224–231. [CrossRef] [PubMed]
8. Hanna, J.N.; Carney, I.K.; Smith, G.A.; Tannenberg, A.E.; Deverill, J.E.; Botha, J.A.; Serafin, I.L.; Harrower, B.J.; Fitzpatrick, P.F.; Searle, J.W. Australian bat lyssavirus infection: A second human case, with a long incubation period. *Med. J. Aust.* **2000**, *172*, 597–599. [PubMed]
9. Australian Technical Advisory Group on Immunisation (ATAGI). Australian Immunisation Handbook. Available online: https://immunisationhandbook.health.gov.au/ (accessed on 14 February 2019).
10. Field, H. The Ecology of Hendra Virus and Australian Bat Lyssavirus. Ph.D. Thesis, University of Queensland, Brisbane, Australia, 2004.
11. Young, M.K.; El Saadi, D.; McCall, B.J. Preventing Australian Bat Lyssavirus: Community knowledge and risk perception of bats in southeast Queensland. *Vector-Borne Zoonotic Dis.* **2014**, *14*, 284–290. [CrossRef] [PubMed]

12. Paterson, B.J.; Butler, M.T.; Eastwood, K.; Cashman, P.M.; Jones, A.; Durrheim, D.N. Cross sectional survey of human-bat interaction in Australia: Public health implications. *BMC Public Health* **2014**, *14*, 58. [CrossRef] [PubMed]

13. Quinn, E.K.; Massey, P.D.; Cox-Witton, K.; Paterson, B.J.; Eastwood, K.; Durrheim, D.N. Understanding human—Bat interactions in NSW, Australia: Improving risk communication for prevention of Australian bat lyssavirus. *BMC Vet. Res.* **2014**, *10*, 144. [CrossRef] [PubMed]

14. McCall, B.J.; Epstein, J.H.; Neill, A.S.; Heel, K.; Field, H.; Barrett, J.; Smith, G.A.; Selvey, L.A.; Rodwell, B.; Lunt, R. Potential exposure to Australian bat lyssavirus, Queensland, 1996-1999. *Emerg. Infect. Dis.* **2000**, *6*, 259–264. [CrossRef] [PubMed]

15. Francis, J.R.; McCall, B.J.; Hutchinson, P.; Powell, J.; Vaska, V.L.; Nourse, C. Australian bat lyssavirus: Implications for public health. *Med. J. Aust.* **2014**, *201*, 647–649. [CrossRef] [PubMed]

16. Churchill, S. *Australian Bats*, 2nd ed.; Allen and Unwin: French Forest, Australia, 1998.

17. Wardell-Johnson, G.; Wardell-Johnson, A.; Bradby, K.; Robinson, T.; Bateman, P.W.; Williams, K.; Keesing, A.; Braun, K.; Beckerling, J.; Burbridge, M. Application of a Gondwanan perspective to restore ecological integrity in the south-western Australian global biodiversity hotspot. *Restor. Ecol.* **2016**, *24*, 805–815. [CrossRef]

18. Smith, I.L.; Northill, J.A.; Harrower, B.J.; Smith, G.A. Detection of Australian bat lyssavirus using a fluorogenic probe. *J. Clin. Virol.* **2002**, *25*, 285–291. [CrossRef]

19. Wadhwa, A.; Wilkins, K.; Gao, J.; Condori Condori, R.E.; Gigante, C.M.; Zhao, H.; Ma, X.; Ellison, J.A.; Greenberg, L.; Velasco-Villa, A.; et al. A Pan-*Lyssavirus* Taqman Real-Time RT-PCR assay for the detection of highly variable rabies *virus* and other lyssaviruses. *PLoS Negl. Trop. Dis.* **2017**, *11*, e0005258. [CrossRef] [PubMed]

20. Rahmadane, I.; Certoma, A.F.; Peck, G.R.; Fitria, Y.; Payne, J.; Colling, A.; Shiell, B.J.; Beddome, G.; Wilson, S.; Yu, M.; et al. Development and validation of an immunoperoxidase antigen detection test for improved diagnosis of rabies in Indonesia. *PLoS Negl. Trop. Dis.* **2017**, *11*, e0006079. [CrossRef] [PubMed]

21. Bossart, K.N.; McEachern, J.A.; Hickey, A.C.; Choudhry, V.; Dimitrov, D.S.; Eaton, B.T.; Wang, L.-F. Neutralization assays for differential henipavirus serology using Bio-Plex Protein Array Systems. *J. Virol. Methods* **2007**, *142*, 29–40. [CrossRef] [PubMed]

22. Hayman, D.T.S.; Suu-Ire, R.; Breed, A.C.; McEachern, J.A.; Wang, L.; Wood, J.L.N.; Cunningham, A.A. Evidence of Henipavirus infection in West African fruit bats. *PLoS ONE* **2008**, *3*, e2739. [CrossRef] [PubMed]

23. Hayman, D.T.S.; Wang, L.-F.; Barr, J.; Baker, K.S.; Suu-Ire, R.; Broder, C.C.; Cunningham, A.A.; Wood, J.L.N. Antibodies to henipavirus or henipa-like viruses in domestic pigs in Ghana, West Africa. *PLoS ONE* **2011**, *6*, e25256. [CrossRef] [PubMed]

24. Plowright, R.K.; Field, H.E.; Smith, C.; Divljan, A.; Palmer, C.; Tabor, G.; Daszak, P.; Foley, J.E. Reproduction and nutritional stress are risk factors for Hendra virus infection in little red flying foxes (*Pteropus scapulatus*). *Proc. R. Soc. B Biol. Sci.* **2008**, *275*, 861–869. [CrossRef] [PubMed]

25. Breed, A.C.; Yu, M.; Barr, J.A.; Crameri, G.; Thalmann, C.M.; Wang, L.F. Prevalence of henipavirus and rubulavirus antibodies in pteropid bats, Papua New Guinea. *Emerg. Infect. Dis.* **2010**, *16*, 1997–1999. [CrossRef] [PubMed]

26. Brown, L.D.; Cai, T.T.; Dasgupta, A. Interval estimation for a binomial proportion. *Stat. Sci.* **2001**, *16*, 101–133. [CrossRef]

27. Aragon, T. *epitools: Epidemiology Tools*, R Package Version 0.5-10; Published 26 October 2017; Available online: https://CRAN.R-project.org/package=epitools (accessed on 21 February 2019).

28. Hammarin, A.L.; Berndtsson, L.T.; Falk, K.; Nedinge, M.; Olsson, G.; Lundkvist, Å. Lyssavirus-reactive antibodies in Swedish bats. *Infect. Ecol. Epidemiol.* **2016**, *6*, 31262. [CrossRef] [PubMed]

29. Wakeley, P.R.; Johnson, N.; McElhinney, L.M.; Marston, D.; Sawyer, J.; Fooks, A.R. Development of a real-time, TaqMan reverse transcription-PCR assay for detection and differentiation of lyssavirus genotypes 1, 5, and 6. *J. Clin. Microbiol.* **2005**, *43*, 2786–2792. [CrossRef] [PubMed]

30. Deubelbeiss, A.; Zahno, M.-L.; Zanoni, M.; Bruegger, D.; Zanoni, R. Real-Time RT-PCR for the detection of lyssavirus species. *J. Vet. Med.* **2014**, *2014*, 476091. [CrossRef] [PubMed]

31. Echevarría, J.E.; Avellón, A.; Juste, J.; Vera, M.; Ibáñez, C. Screening of active lyssavirus infection in wild bat populations by viral RNA detection on oropharyngeal swabs. *J. Clin. Microbiol.* **2001**, *39*, 3678–3683. [CrossRef] [PubMed]

32. Amengual, B.; Bourhy, H.; López-Roig, M.; Serra-Cobo, J. Temporal dynamics of European bat lyssavirus type 1 and survival of Myotis myotis bats in natural colonies. *PLoS ONE* **2007**, *2*, e566. [CrossRef] [PubMed]
33. Franka, R.; Johnson, N.; Muller, T.; Vos, A.; Neubert, L.; Freuling, C.; Rupprecht, C.E.; Fooks, A.R. Susceptibility of North American big brown bats (*Eptesicus fuscus*) to infection with European bat lyssavirus type 1. *J. Gen. Virol.* **2008**, *89*, 1998–2010. [CrossRef] [PubMed]
34. Shankar, V.; Bowen, R.A.; Davis, A.D.; Rupprecht, C.E.; O'Shea, T.J. Rabies in a captive colony of big brown bats (*Eptesicus fuscus*). *J. Wildl. Dis.* **2004**, *40*, 403–413. [CrossRef] [PubMed]

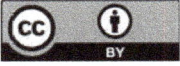

Tropical Medicine and Infectious Disease

MDPI

Brief Report

A Short Report on the Lack of a Pyrogenic Response of Australian Genomic Group IV Isolates of *Coxiella burnetii* in Guinea Pigs

Aminul Islam [1,*], John Stenos [1], Gemma Vincent [1] and Stephen Graves [1,2]

[1]   Australian Rickettsial Reference Laboratory, University Hospital Geelong, Geelong, VIC 3220, Australia;
      johns@barwonhealth.org.au (J.S.); gvince@barwonhealth.org.au (G.V.); graves.rickettsia@gmail.com (S.G.)
[2]   New South Wales Health Pathology, Nepean Hospital, Penrith, NSW 2751, Australia
*   Correspondence: aislam.islam@gmail.com; Tel.: +61-(0)-402-387-013

Received: 30 December 2018; Accepted: 23 January 2019; Published: 25 January 2019

Abstract: This small study reports on a non-pyrogenic response of five different Australian isolates of *Coxiella burnetii* (*C. burnetii*). They were all members of Genomic Group IV and obtained from three cases of acute human infection, one case of chronic human infection and one case of goat abortion. The guinea pigs infected with these isolates did not develop fever (temperature $\geq 40.0\,^{\circ}\text{C}$), which is consistent with other members of this genomic group that were isolated from elsewhere in the world. In contrast, guinea pigs infected with the classical USA tick isolate, Nine Mile phase 1 (RSA 493) of Genomic Group I, experienced a four-day febrile period.

Keywords: *C. burnetii*; Q fever; Australia; pyrogenicity; guinea pigs

1. Introduction

Guinea pigs are an excellent small animal model of acute Q fever (infection with *Coxiella burnetii* or *C. burnetii*) in humans [1–3]. However, not all isolates of *C. burnetii* will cause fever (pyrogenicity) in guinea pigs. This feature of the bacterium appears to be related to the genomic group to which the isolate belongs, with group IV and VI known to be non-pyrogenic [4].

Recent Australian isolates of *C. burnetii* belong to a unique subset of genomic group IV; however, most were isolated from patients with acute Q fever, many of whom had presented with fever [5]. The question investigated in this small study was whether a selection of these Australian isolates were pyrogenic in guinea pigs.

2. Materials and Methods

2.1. Animal Ethics

This study was approved by the Australian Rickettsial Reference Laboratory Animal Care and Ethics Committee (ACEC/010). All experimental works were performed in a biosafety level 3 laboratory at the Department of Microbiology, John Hunter Hospital, Newcastle, New South Wales, Australia.

2.2. Coxiella Burnetii Isolates

Five Australian isolates of *C. burnetii* were selected for use in this study, with a range of molecular and epidemiological features (Table 1). All were members of genomic group IV, but represented three different genotypes (CbAu01, CbAu04 and CbAu06) according to a multi-locus variable number of tandem repeats (VNTR) analysis (MLVA). These genotypes were shown to be unique to Australia [5]. There were four human isolates that came from three cases of acute infection (AuQ01, AuQ10 and

AuQ43) and one case of chronic infection (AuQ04). There was also one isolate from an aborting goat (AuQ57), which was associated with a number of human cases [6].

C. *burnetii* Nine Mile phase 1 (RSA493), originally obtained from a tick in the USA and belonging to Genomic Group I, was used as a positive control, as it was known to be pyrogenic in guinea pigs. Sterile cell culture medium (RPMI-1640) was used as a negative control.

Table 1. Brief molecular and epidemiological features of the five Australian isolates of *Coxiella burnetii* (*C. burnetii*) used in the pyrogenicity study.

C. *burnetii* Isolates	MLVA * Genotype	Epidemiological Features						
		Type of Q Fever	Year	Location	Animal Contact	Symptoms	Source of Isolate
AuQ01 (Human)	CbAu01	Acute	2005	Armidale, Northern NSW	Goat	Fever, Jaundice	Blood
AuQ04 (Human)	CbAu04	Chronic	2007	Swan Hill, Northern VIC	Unknown	Fever, Endocarditis/ Aortic valve incompetence	Surgically removed tissue
AuQ10 (Human)	CbAu06	Acute	2011	Coffs Harbour, Northern NSW	Unknown	Fever, Haemophagocytic Syndrome	Blood
AuQ43 (Human)	CbAu01	Acute	2012	Mt Louisa, Northern QLD	Unknown	Fever	Blood
AuQ57 (Animal)	CbAu01	Goat coxiello-sis	2012	Meredith, Central VIC	Goat	Abortion	Aborted foetus

* MLVA-multiple locus variable number of tandem repeats analysis.

2.3. Culture and Quantification of C. burnetii in VERO Cell Line and Wild Mice

Vero cells were grown in 10ml RPMI (Gibco, Australia) supplemented with 10% new born calf serum (NBCS) (Gibco, Australia) and 1% L-glutamine (Gibco, Australia). The five C. *burnetii* isolates were inoculated into Vero cell monolayer and grown at 37 °C with 5% CO_2 for 14 days. The infected monolayer was removed by scrapping and each preparation inoculated intraperitoneally into a single outbred mouse. This was done to ensure that all C. *burnetii* cells were in phase 1 (virulent) for the later guinea pig infection [7]. Each infected mouse was euthanized seven days later and its enlarged spleen removed aseptically. Each spleen was separately homogenized in 5 mL of Hank's Balanced Salt Solution and the concentration of C. *burnetii* DNA measured by quantitative real-time PCR (qPCR) using an assay targeting the single-copy com1 gene [8]. Each spleen suspension was adjusted to contain between 10^6 and 10^7 C. *burnetii* per 0.2 mL.

2.4. Experimental Guinea Pig Infection

Outbred breeds of adult male guinea pigs were used in this study (*n* = 24). One week prior to the start of the experiment, an IPTT300 temperature transponder (Biomedic Data Systems, Inc., Seaford, DE, USA) was implanted into the sub-cutaneous tissue on the flank of each guinea pig.

Each guinea pig was anaesthetized with a 0.2 mL intramuscular injection of 9.5 mL of ketamine (100 mg/mL) and 0.5 mL of xylazine (100 mg/mL). Each anaesthetized guinea pig had 0.2 mL of the infected mouse spleen suspension introduced slowly into its nostrils via a fine-bore plastic Pasteur pipette. The guinea pigs inhaled the liquid slowly and the C. *burnetii* presumably entered the animals' lungs.

2.5. Monitoring Guinea Pig Temperature with Probe

Guinea pig temperatures were recorded daily for 21 days using an IPTT-300 Smart Probe held over the location of the subcutaneous temperature transponder in the guinea pig.

A temperature at or above 40 °C was defined as a fever and the guinea pig considered to be febrile. The experiment was terminated at day 21 post-infection by which time all guinea pig temperatures had returned to normal.

3. Results

The temperature changes in the 24 guinea pigs (grouped according to the isolate of *C. burnetii* used to infect them) are shown in the Figure 1. The four guinea pigs given only Roswell Park Memorial Institute (RPMI) medium intranasally (negative controls) did not develop a fever at any stage.

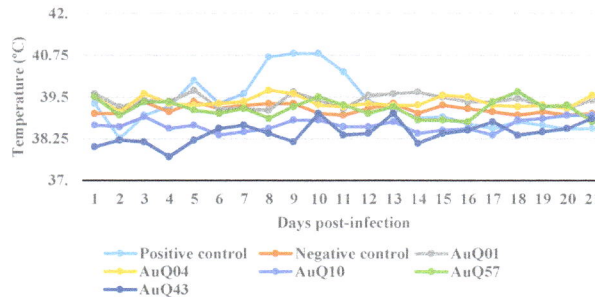

Figure 1. The temperature pattern of guinea pigs infected with five different Australian isolates of *C. burnetii*, with the positive (NM1) and negative (sterile RPMI 1640 media) controls over a period of 21 days post-infection. Febrile response (temperature ≥ 40.0 °C) in positive controls sustained from days 8–11 with an early onset at day 5. Throughout the experimental period, the five Australian isolates and negative control did not show febrile response and remained under 40.0 °C. The average value of temperature in each group is shown in the graph.

The four guinea pigs given *C. burnetii* Nine Mile phase 1 (positive control), developed fever (40.6 ± 0.3) from days 8–11 after infection (four-day duration). None of the five Australian *C. burnetii* isolates, inoculated into 16 guinea pigs, resulted in fever (38.6 ± 1.0). They were all non-pyrogenic.

4. Discussion

The best small animal model for studying Q fever is the guinea pig, as it develops a fever of limited duration, similar to infected humans [3]. However, not all isolates of *C. burnetii* are pyrogenic in the guinea pig. Studies of non-Australian isolates show that those from genomic groups IV and VI are non-pyrogenic [4]. This study has now demonstrated the same phenomenon of non-pyrogenicity in five Australian isolates, which all belong to genomic group IV, albeit to a unique subgroup. The four human isolates used in this study caused fever in the human patients from whom the bacteria were obtained. However, they did not cause fever in the guinea pigs. While the pathological basis for this difference is not known, there is a practical significance to it. When using guinea pigs to test new vaccines for use against Q fever and using abrogation of fever as a clinical indicator of vaccine success, it is necessary to use a challenge isolate of *C. burnetii* that causes fever in the non-immunized guinea pigs. On the basis of this small study it will not be possible to use Australian isolates of *C. burnetii* for challenge in Q fever vaccine studies, if abrogation of fever is used as a clinical marker of vaccine protection. It appears that the Nine Mile phase 1 isolate of *C. burnetii* is required for this purpose.

5. Conclusions

Australian isolates of *C. burnetii* do not cause fever in experimentally infected guinea pigs, confirming what has been shown in other genomic group IV isolates elsewhere in the world.

Trop. Med. Infect. Dis. **2019**, *4*, 18

Author Contributions: A.I., G.V. and S.G. designed and carried out the experiments. J.S. provided scientific guidance and administrative support.

Funding: This research received no external funding.

Acknowledgments: The financial support of Anne Crotty and the administrative support of Stephen Braye, both of NSW Health Pathology, Newcastle, Australia, is appreciated.

Conflicts of Interest: The authors declare no conflict of interests.

References

1. Scott, G.H.; Burger, G.T.; Kishimoto, R.A. Experimental *Coxiella burnetii* infection of guinea pigs and mice. *Lab. Anim. Sci.* **1978**, *28*, 673–675. [PubMed]
2. Russell-Lodrigue, K.E.; Zhang, G.Q.; McMurray, D.N.; Samuel, J.E. Clinical and pathologic changes in a guinea pig aerosol challenge model of acute Q fever. *Infect. Immun.* **2006**, *74*, 6085–6091. [CrossRef] [PubMed]
3. Bewley, K.R. Animal models of Q fever (*Coxiella burnetii*). *Comp. Med.* **2013**, *63*, 469–476.
4. Russell-Lodrigue, K.E.; Andoh, M.; Poels, W.J.; Shive, H.R.; Weeks, B.R.; Zhang, G.Q.; Tersteeg, C.; Masegi, T.; Hotta, A.; Yamaguchi, Y.; et al. *Coxiella burnetii* isolates cause genogroup-specific virulence in mice and guinea pig models of acute Q fever. *Infect. Immun.* **2009**, *77*, 5640–5650. [CrossRef] [PubMed]
5. Vincent, G.; Stenos, J.; Latham, J.; Fenwick, S.; Graves, S. Novel genotypes of *Coxiella burnetii* identified in isolates from Australian Q fever patients. *Int. J Med. Micro.* **2016**, *306*, 463–470. [CrossRef]
6. Bond, K.A.; Vincent, G.; Wilks, C.R.; Franklin, L.; Sutton, B.; Stenos, J.; Cowan, R.; Lim, K.; Athan, E.; Harris, O.; et al. One health approach to controlling a Q fever outbreak on an Australian goat farm. *Epidemiol. Infect.* **2016**, *144*, 1129–1141. [CrossRef]
7. Ormsbee, R.A.; Bell, E.J.; Lackman, D.B.; Tallent, G. The influence of phase on the protective potency of Q fever vaccine. *J. Immunol.* **1964**, *92*, 404–412. [PubMed]
8. Lockhart, M.G.; Graves, S.R.; Banazis, M.J.; Fenwick, S.G.; Stenos, J. A comparison of methods for extracting DNA from *Coxiella burnetii* as measured by a duplex qPCR assay. *Lett. Appl. Microbiol.* **2011**, *52*, 513–520. [CrossRef] [PubMed]

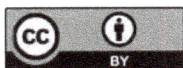

*Tropical Medicine and
Infectious Disease*

MDPI

Review

Japanese Encephalitis Virus in Australia: From Known Known to Known Unknown

Andrew F. van den Hurk [1,*], Alyssa T. Pyke [1], John S. Mackenzie [2], Sonja Hall-Mendelin [1] and Scott A. Ritchie [3]

1 Public Health Virology, Forensic and Scientific Services, Department of Health, Queensland Government, PO Box 594, Archerfield, QLD 4108, Australia; Alyssa.Pyke@health.qld.gov.au (A.T.P.); Sonja.Hall-Mendelin@health.qld.gov.au (S.H.-M.)
2 Faculty of Medical Sciences, Curtin University, and Division of Microbiology and Infectious Diseases, PathWest, Locked Bag2009, Nedlands, WA 6909, Australia; J.Mackenzie@curtin.edu.au
3 College of Public Health, Medical and Veterinary Sciences, and Australian Institute of Tropical Health and Medicine, James Cook University, PO Box 6811, Cairns, QLD 4870, Australia; scott.ritchie@jcu.edu.au
* Correspondence: andrew.vandenhurk@health.qld.gov.au; Tel.: +61-7-3096-2858

Received: 23 January 2019; Accepted: 19 February 2019; Published: 20 February 2019

Abstract: Japanese encephalitis virus (JEV) is a major cause of neurological disease in Asia. It is a zoonotic flavivirus transmitted between water birds and/or pigs by *Culex* mosquitoes; humans are dead-end hosts. In 1995, JEV emerged for the first time in northern Australia causing an unprecedented outbreak in the Torres Strait. In this article, we revisit the history of JEV in Australia and describe investigations of JEV transmission cycles in the Australian context. Public health responses to the incipient outbreak included vaccination and sentinel pig surveillance programs. Virus isolation and vector competence experiments incriminated *Culex annulirostris* as the likely regional vector. The role this species plays in transmission cycles depends on the availability of domestic pigs as a blood source. Experimental evidence suggests that native animals are relatively poor amplifying hosts of JEV. The persistence and predominantly annual virus activity between 1995 and 2005 suggested that JEV had become endemic in the Torres Strait. However, active surveillance was discontinued at the end of 2005, so the status of JEV in northern Australia is unknown. Novel mosquito-based surveillance systems provide a means to investigate whether JEV still occurs in the Torres Strait or is no longer a risk to Australia.

Keywords: Japanese encephalitis virus; zoonosis; mosquito; transmission; Australia

1. Introduction

Japanese encephalitis virus (JEV) is a single-strand, positive-sense RNA virus of the genus *Flavivirus*, family *Flaviviridae*. The virus is responsible for approximately 68,000 clinical cases annually and is the leading cause of encephalitis in a number of countries in Southeast Asia, the Indian sub-continent and the Indonesian archipelago [1]. Predominantly asymptomatic, less than 1% of human infections result in clinical disease which can range broadly in severity from a mild febrile illness to acute meningomyeloencephalitis. Of symptomatic cases, 20–30% are fatal, and among the survivors, approximately 30–50% will have ongoing neurological sequelae.

Prevalent in tropical and subtropical parts of Asia and the Pacific rim [2], JEV exists in a zoonotic transmission cycle between ardeid wading birds, such as herons and egrets, and *Culex* mosquitoes, particularly, *Culex tritaeniorhynchus* and *Cx. vishnui* which utilize rice fields for larval development [3]. Domestic pigs are important amplifying hosts, due to rates of infection of 90–100%, development of viremia levels sufficient to infect mosquitoes and constant annual turnover leading to a continual supply of immunologically naïve pigs as susceptible hosts. Recent experiments have demonstrated that JEV can be transmitted directly between pigs via oronasal secretions further enhancing the status of pigs as amplifying hosts [4]. Although the epidemiological significance of this finding needs to be definitively established, it suggests that virus transmission can potentially occur in the absence of suitable mosquito vectors. Humans and horses can develop fatal disease, but they are considered dead end hosts of JEV because they do not produce adequate viral levels required to infect mosquitoes. Thus, JEV is considered an important zoonotic pathogen and a concerted One Health approach is required for sustained disease suppression [5].

In Australia, JEV is mostly viewed as an issue for travelers to endemic regions and occasional overseas acquired cases are reported [6–8]. However, in 1995, JEV was first recognized in natural transmission cycles in northern Australia when a widespread outbreak occurred on the islands of the Torres Strait, the body of water that separates Cape York Peninsula and the New Guinea landmass (Figure 1). Three human cases, two of which were fatal, occurred on the island of Badu. This event was unprecedented, as Murray Valley encephalitis virus (MVEV) and West Nile virus Kunjin subtype (WNV$_{KUN}$) were considered the only encephalitogenic flaviviruses southeast of Wallacea, the region that separates the Asian and Australasian zoogeographical regions. In the current paper, we revisit the epidemiology of JEV in the Australasian region and summarize research conducted to elucidate the factors that led to its emergence and apparent disappearance.

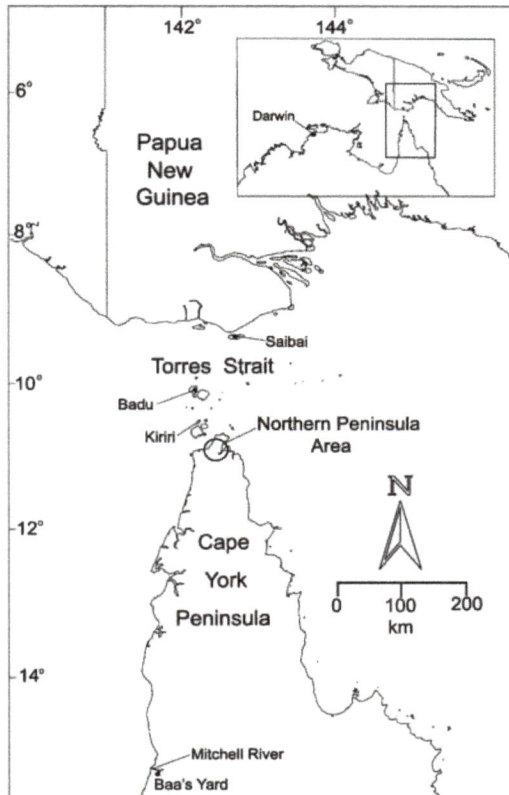

Figure 1. Map of Northern Australia and southern Papua New Guinea showing locations mentioned in the text. The Northern Peninsula Area includes the communities of Bamaga, Injinoo, New Mapoon, Seisia, and Umagico.

2. The Emergence of JEV in Northern Australia

In March 1995, Public Health authorities were notified of three cases of encephalitis on Badu in the Torres Strait [9]. Given previous MVEV activity in northern Australia, it was initially suspected that this virus was the etiological agent. However, virus isolation from serum samples from two asymptomatic residents of the island and mosquitoes yielded JEV isolates. Several other residents and domestic pigs were also found to be JEV seropositive by enzyme linked immunosorbent assay (ELISA) and hemagglutination inhibition (HAI) assay. Whilst it is known that flavivirus cross-reactivity can obscure serological findings and complicate result interpretation, a proportion of these serum samples also demonstrated specific neutralizing antibodies at notably higher titers to JEV than to MVEV or WNV$_{KUN}$, providing further definitive evidence that JEV had caused the outbreak [9]. Virus genotyping revealed that the Badu 1995 human and mosquito isolates clustered within genotype II [9]. *Culex annulirostris* was the only mosquito that yielded JEV at a carriage rate of 2.97 per 1000 mosquitoes, indicating that this was the potential mosquito vector [10]. Subsequent, broader serosurveys of humans and pigs revealed that the outbreak was widespread across the Torres Strait, although Badu appeared to have conditions conducive to epizootic JEV transmission. This included an immunologically naïve human population and a large immunologically naïve domestic pig population, with numerous pigpens located close to houses. There were also widespread productive larval habitats of *Cx. annulirostris*, created by poorly maintained drains, damaged septic systems, and groundwater sites which had become nutrient rich due to feces from horses that had been introduced to the island in the year preceding the outbreak [11]. Emergency vector control strategies included treatment of larval sites with the insect growth regulator, *s*-methoprene, and thermal fogging of adults with the pyrethroid, bioresmethrin.

Following this incipient outbreak, several strategies were employed to limit JEV transmission, both on Badu and on other islands. A vaccination program using the formalin inactivated mouse brain-derived vaccine (Biken Institute, Japan) commenced in December 1995 and by March 1996, 93% of residents of the outer islands who commenced the schedule had received at least 2 doses [12]. To detect further JEV activity, a sentinel pig program was established on 4 islands of the Torres Strait, as well as proximal to mainland Australian communities on the tip of Cape York Peninsula [13]. To reduce the availability of larval habitats, maintenance and drainage works were initiated on Badu, although the swampy ground present over much of the island limited the impact of this strategy on adult mosquito populations [11]. In 1996 and 1997, JEV activity, as evidenced by seroconversions of sentinel pigs, appeared restricted to the northernmost island of Saibai.

The unexpected emergence of JEV in the Australasian region prompted investigations of the origins of the virus and potential mechanisms of introduction. Between 1996 and 1998, almost 400,000 mosquitoes were processed from the Western Province of Papua New Guinea (PNG) yielding 3 isolates [14]. Furthermore, there was evidence of human infection in PNG, as demonstrated by JEV-specific antibodies in sera collected as far back as 1989 [15] and by clinical cases of encephalitis (J Oakley and S. Flew, unpublished data cited by [14]. Thus, it appeared that the New Guinea landmass was the source of the incursions. Furthermore, backtrack simulations by Ritchie and Rochester [16] suggested that wind-borne mosquitoes carried by low pressure systems from New Guinea could have been the mechanism of virus introduction.

In 1998, widespread JEV activity again occurred in the Torres Strait and, for the first time, on the Australian mainland [17]. There were two clinical human cases recognized serologically during this outbreak, with the first being in an unvaccinated child on Badu and the second being a fisherman at the mouth of the Mitchell River on western Cape York Peninsula. Sentinel pigs on many outer islands seroconverted to the virus, whilst seroconversion of pigs on Kiriri Island signaled the first evidence of transmission occurring on the inner Torres Strait islands. On the mainland, sentinel pigs on the Northern Peninsula Area (NPA) and at Baa's Yard near the Mitchell River, seroconverted to JEV, and the virus was isolated from 3 pigs at Seisia on the NPA. Collections on Badu yielded 42 isolates of JEV from 31,898 mosquitoes, with all but one coming from *Cx. sitiens* subgroup mosquitoes (primarily *Cx.*

annulirostris); the other isolate was from *Aedes vigilax* [18]. In contrast, no JEV was detected in 35,235 mosquitoes processed from the Australian mainland [19]. Nucleotide sequence analysis and molecular genotyping of mosquito and pig 1998 isolates revealed that they also belonged to genotype II. A high nucleotide identity was also demonstrated between the sequences of the 1998 and 1995 Torres Strait viruses, and to the Australian mainland and PNG sequences, highly suggesting that the origin of JEV incursions into Northern Australia may have been PNG [17,18]. Following the 1998 outbreak, and with a view to reducing contact and transmission between pigs, mosquitoes, and humans, domestic pigs were relocated from proximal to houses to communal pig pens >2 km away from the community.

The magnitude of the 1998 outbreak of JEV in the Torres Strait and Cape York Peninsula was unprecedented in both spatial scale and intensity. JEV activity was recorded from southern PNG, across most of the Torres Strait and south to western Cape York Peninsula [14,17], suggesting a unique and extreme event. The outbreak appeared to represent the convergence of high populations of *Culex* mosquitoes and widespread JEV transmission in southern PNG, coupled with a strong tropical cyclone in the Gulf of Carpentaria that may have transported JEV infected mosquitoes from PNG into the Torres Strait and deep into Cape York Peninsula. Late 1997 to early 1998 featured a strong *El-Nino* event that caused severe drought in the Western Province of PNG [20]. Normally flooded wetlands may have been reduced to stagnant pools of highly organic water favorable for the production of *Cx. sitiens* subgroup mosquitoes. Indeed, mosquito collections in February 1998 in Western Province were very high, with many traps catching over 10,000 mosquitoes per night [16], from which JEV was isolated [14]. This event was also coupled with the occurrence of Tropical Cyclone Sid in the western Gulf of Carpentaria in late December 1997. The large wind field of this category 2 cyclone was potentially sufficient to transport mosquitoes from southern New Guinea to west central Cape York Peninsula, where JEV activity occurred at the mouth of the Mitchell River [16]. The coincidental occurrence of two extreme events, drought induced JEV transmission in southern PNG and a cyclone in the Gulf of Carpentaria that could transport the mosquitoes from New Guinea landmass deep into the Cape York Peninsula, make a repeat of this event unlikely.

After no recognized activity in 1999, JEV reappeared in the Torres Strait in 2000. Although virus was not isolated from 7652 *Cx. annulirostris* collected from Badu, a single JEV isolate was obtained from 84 *Cx. gelidus* mosquitoes [21]. Collections from Saibai Island also yielded an isolate, albeit from *Cx. sitiens* subgroup mosquitoes [22]. JEV isolates were also obtained from the acute sera of three pigs on Badu. Interestingly, molecular genotyping of the two mosquito and pig sera 2000 isolates demonstrated they belonged to genotype I and did not cluster with the previous Australian 1995 and 1998 genotype II viruses. Importantly, this demonstrated the introduction of a new JEV genotype into Australia and highlighted the continued risk and vulnerability of the region to further JEV incursions [22,23].

Between 2001 and 2005, sentinel pigs and/or deployment of a newly developed remote mosquito trapping system were effective in detection of JEV on Badu Island every year [24]. In 2004, the virus was again detected on mainland Australia, when pigs located on the NPA seroconverted to JEV and a single isolate was obtained from a pool of *Cx. sitiens* subgroup mosquitoes collected from the Bamaga rubbish dump [25]. This was the first time that JEV had been isolated from mosquitoes collected from the Australian mainland. Molecular phylogenetic analysis revealed that the virus clustered with a 2004 Badu pig isolate, and 2000 mosquito and pig sequences in genotype I. As no further evidence of genotype II in the region had been demonstrated since 1998, these findings suggested this genotype may have been subsequently replaced by genotype I.

The sentinel pig program and remote mosquito trapping trials were discontinued in the Torres Strait at the end of the 2005, whilst the sentinel pigs were removed from the NPA in 2011. However, given the continual risk of re-emergence, in 2012, mosquito-based surveillance was re-deployed, albeit using a different system (refer to Section 3.3) in the NPA by the Northern Australia Quarantine Service. Despite multiple detections of MVEV and WNV$_{KUN}$ in the NPA traps which were most notable in 2015 [26], there has been no evidence of recent JEV activity (T. Kerlin and K. Rickart, unpublished data). Traps were also run on Badu, but only during the 2012–2013 wet season. No JEV was detected during this period of deployment. Thus, the status of JEV in the Torres Strait since 2005 is unknown.

3. Elucidating the Ecology of JEV Transmission Cycles in Australia

3.1. Vertebrate Host Studies

Numerous vertebrate species have been investigated as amplifying hosts of JEV in endemic regions, although ardeid birds and pigs are considered the most important [2]. When JEV appeared in northern Australia, it was feared that the large populations of feral pigs and wading birds on the mainland would provide an abundance of amplifying hosts to allow the virus to become established in natural transmission cycles. An unknown quantity and continuing concern is the role that other vertebrates, particularly native species, could play in these transmission cycles. Unfortunately, laboratory based vertebrate studies are very complex, requiring high level biocontainment, which restricts them to a limited number of laboratories in Australia. Thus, there has only been limited experimentation on the course of JEV infection in Australian vertebrates. In experiments conducted well before JEV emerged in Australia, the Nankeen Night Heron, *Nycticorax caledonicus*, was shown to produce viremia levels that could potentially infect recipient mosquitoes [27]. Later, the response of marsupials to JEV infection was investigated at the Australian Animal Health Laboratories (AAHL). It was shown that eastern grey kangaroos, agile wallabies and tammar wallabies either did not develop detectable viremia or were only capable of producing viremia levels below the threshold required to infect questing mosquitoes (PW Daniels, D Middleton, D Boyle, K Newberry, D Williams, R Lunt, unpublished data cited by Mackenzie et al. [28]). In contrast, possums produced a higher viremia when compared to the macropods tested. The only other native species examined as a potential amplifying host in laboratory-based experiments was the black flying fox, *Pteropus alecto* [29]. Only 1 of 15 flying foxes produced a detectable viremia which was sufficient to infect recipient mosquitoes. Interestingly, 3 other flying foxes were able to infect recipient mosquitoes, even though they did not produce a viremia that was detectable using a highly sensitive real-time reverse transcriptase PCR. Despite exhibiting low infection rates following experimental exposure, flying foxes could still play a role in the ecology of JEV in Northern Australia, as they roost in camps containing 1000s of individuals, are prevalent on a number of islands of the Torres Strait and are known to migrate from the New Guinea landmass.

The importance of pigs as amplifying hosts of JEV and the existence of large, abundant feral populations across Northern Australia prompted pig infection studies with a regional context. Of particular interest, was whether prior exposure to endemic MVEV or WNV$_{KUN}$ viruses affected pig susceptibility to JEV infection and how this may impact on their immune responses. In experiments performed at AAHL, JEV was readily detected in pigs following primary JEV infection, but not in pigs previously infected with MVEV or WNV$_{KUN}$ that were later challenged with JEV [30]. Coupled with suppressed JEV viremia levels, elevation of existing cross-reactive JEV neutralizing antibodies were further demonstrated in these pigs. Notably, these findings suggest that prior exposure to MVEV or WNV$_{KUN}$ may elicit protective immunity against JEV in pigs. Together with the suppression of viremia levels, this indicates that pre-immune pigs may not be effective amplifying hosts and therefore are unlikely to play a major role in JEV transmission.

3.2. Incrimination of Mosquito Vectors

In the majority of regions where JEV is known to circulate, *Cx. tritaeniorhynchus* and *Cx. vishnui* are the key mosquito vectors, however, these species, do not occur in Northern Australia. Based on its role as the primary vector of MVEV and WNV$_{KUN}$ [31], it was suspected that an alternate species, *Cx. annulirostris*, was the primary vector during the original Torres Strait 1995 outbreak. This hypothesis was further supported by the fact that this was the only species from which JEV isolates were recovered during this initial outbreak and to date, has been the species yielding the most isolates obtained in Northern Australia. Subsequent laboratory-based vector competence experiments using genotype II JEV isolated from Badu Island in 1998 confirmed the status of *Cx. annulirostris* as the likely primary vector in Australia [32]. Interestingly, Hemmerter et al. [33] demonstrated that *Cx. annulirostris* contains at least 5 mitochondrial cytochrome oxidase I lineages, with some having a wide distribution in the Australasian regions, whilst others appeared more restricted geographically. It was revealed that three of these lineages occurred in southern PNG, the Torres Strait and Cape York Peninsula. The authors hypothesized that these lineages may vary in their vector competence for JEV, thus potentially explaining the southern limits of the virus on the Australian mainland. Phenotypic evidence to corroborate this hypothesis was provided by Johnson et al. [34] who showed that the dominant mainland Australian lineage of *Cx. annulirostris* was a relatively poor laboratory vector of the genotype I JEV.

Studies of other species which yielded isolates demonstrated that *Cx. gelidus* was a highly efficient laboratory vector [34] whereas *Ae. vigilax* had a comparatively low transmission rate [32]. Although other species, such as *Cx. sitiens* and *Cx. quinquefasciatus* were efficient laboratory vectors [32] and have been implicated as secondary vectors in SE Asia, their status as vectors in Northern Australia remains largely unknown. Finally, electrophoretic analysis of collections of *Cx. annulirostris* that yielded JEV revealed that the closely related and morphologically similar *Cx. palpalis* was present, sometimes at high levels [35]. Thus, this species could also be considered a potential JEV vector. Similar to the situation in endemic locations, the evidence from virus detection in field collected mosquitoes and vector competence experiments incriminates members of the genus *Culex* as the primary vectors of JEV in Northern Australia.

3.3. The Influence of Mosquito Host Feeding Patterns on JEV Transmission in Northern Australia

The propensity for the mosquito to feed on the vertebrate host is critical to its role as a virus vector. Analysis of host feeding patterns of *Cx. annulirostris* from numerous locations in northern Australia revealed that, for the most part, pigs and birds accounted for only a small percentage of positive blood meals [36,37]. Instead, most of the blood meals obtained by *Cx. annulirostris* originated from marsupials, particularly the Agile Wallaby, *Macropus agilis* [37,38]. As mentioned previously, experiments conducted at AAHL had previously shown that Agile wallabies produced only low-level viremia. Thus, predilection for *Cx. annulirostris* to feed on wallabies may have dampened transmission, particularly on the mainland, by diverting host seeking mosquitoes away from pigs. Interestingly, there are no wallabies on Badu, so this possible dampening effect would not have impacted transmission dynamics on the island.

The only locations where significant feeding on pigs was recorded in northern Australia was from locations adjacent to domestic pigs or where feral pigs congregated, such as rubbish dumps. In endemic areas in Southeast Asia, intense JEV transmission is usually driven by pig feeding rates >30%. Thus, it was not surprising when analysis of *Cx. annulirostris* host feeding patterns during periods of recognized JEV transmission also revealed relatively high porcine feeding rates, as high as 80% [36,37]. The proportion of *Cx. annulirostris* feeding on pigs was significantly reduced when the domestic pigs were relocated from the Badu community to a communal piggery some 2.5 km away [21]. However, this did not appear to eliminate virus transmission close to human habitation, as infected mosquitoes were subsequently collected within the community [39], although it may have diminished the potential for transmission. It was suggested that domestic pigs needed to be moved further away to be out of the flight range of *Cx. annulirostris*, which can be as much as 12 km [40].

3.4. Development of Mosquito-Based JEV Surveillance Systems

Undoubtedly, the sentinel pig surveillance program played a considerable role in providing evidence of JEV activity and, in some cases, seroconversion in herds preceded human cases [17]. However, the use of sentinel pigs for detection of viral activity has several limitations affecting their continued deployment, particularly in remote areas [24]. Firstly, the fact that pigs are a key amplifying host of the virus is an obvious risk which may exacerbate and contribute to ongoing transmission. Secondly, sentinel animal programs can be highly expensive to establish and maintain, impacting on local resources and resulting in a major financial burden to biosecurity and public health authorities. Efficient running and effectiveness of sentinel animal programs may also be affected by labor-intensive bleeding and collection procedures which can lead to occupational health and safety issues and, if delayed, can greatly affect downstream result interpretation and disease management strategies. The inherent difficulty in distinguishing JEV from MVEV and WNV_{KUN} infections in serological assays due to cross-reacting antibodies may also obscure accurate laboratory interpretations and require further testing by highly specialized reference laboratories [30].

A surveillance system involving detection of viral RNA in mosquitoes collected in continuously run mosquito traps has been developed as an alternative to using sentinel pigs. The original iterations of this mosquito-based system involved processing all mosquitoes collected in solar or propane-powered traps [24]. However, these traps had the capacity to collect >150,000 mosquitoes in a week, so diagnostic capacity was overwhelmed. To circumvent the need to process hundreds of pools, a system was developed that takes advantage of the sugar feeding behavior of mosquitoes [41]. In this system, mosquitoes are collected in CO_2-baited traps, where they can feed on honey-soaked nucleic acid preservation cards, which are submitted for detection of viral RNA [42]. A number of modifications have been made to the trapping system, resulting in the current trap design, the sentinel mosquito arbovirus capture kit (SMACK) which does not require electricity and maximizes survivability of collected mosquitoes, thus increasing the likelihood of multiple feedings on the cards [26,43].

The sugar-based arbovirus system has been trialled in several locations around Australia and has detected a number of arboviruses, including MVEV and WNV_{KUN}, the alphaviruses, Ross River and Barmah Forest viruses, and the bunyavirus Gan Gan [26,42,44,45]. Detection of WNV_{KUN} in traps deployed near Darwin, Northern Territory, without concurrent detection in sentinel chickens demonstrated that the system is potentially more sensitive than sentinel animals in some instances [45]. Furthermore, if enough viral RNA is expectorated on the cards, it can provide a template for nucleotide gene sequencing in phylogenetic studies. The sugar-based arbovirus system using SMACK traps is now deployed operationally at 12 remote locations in Queensland, including communities in the NPA. Although JEV has not been detected in cards removed from field-deployed traps, results from laboratory-based studies showed that this virus could readily be detected in saliva expectorated by sugar-feeding mosquitoes [41]. This indicates that the sugar-based system has direct utility for JEV surveillance.

In the current sugar-based arbovirus system, the small amounts of virus expectorated on the nucleic acid preservation cards means that some samples deemed positive are at the limit of detection in molecular assays [45]. To increase the sensitivity of the sugar-based surveillance system for arbovirus detection, investigations are currently underway into the utility of mosquito excreta as an alternative sample type to saliva [46]. Early results have demonstrated that both WNV_{KUN} and dengue viruses can be detected in excreta at a higher rate than it is detected in the saliva, and possibly represents the greater volume of liquid excreted by mosquitoes (1.5 µL) compared with the volume of saliva expectorated (4.7 nL) [46,47].

4. Conclusions

To date, the detection of JEV in mosquitoes collected in a mosquito trap on Badu in March 2005 signified the final time that virus activity was unequivocally detected in Northern Australia. Overall, the virus was detected in 10 out of 11 years between 1995 and 2005 indicating that JEV had either become established in enzootic cycles in the Torres Strait or was re-introduced during the period almost annually when conditions were suitable.

Despite the status of the JEV in the Torres Strait being largely unknown, the ongoing vaccination program has likely limited the number of human cases. The vaccines currently utilized in the Torres Strait are the live attenuated, recombinant vaccine (IMOJEV) and the inactivated, African green monkey kidney (Vero) cell culture-derived vaccine (JEspect) [48]. Vaccination is recommended for residents of the outer islands and non-residents who spend a cumulative total of 30 days in the Torres Strait during the wet season (December to May) and, as such, is offered as part of an immunization program in risk areas.

The lack of evidence of JEV activity on Badu since 2005 likely represents limited surveillance rather than natural disappearance of the virus from the region. Human infection with JEV resulting in clinical disease is rigorously investigated and is defined as clinical evidence of non-encephalitic and encephalitic disease coupled with definitive laboratory testing [49]. However, the majority of JEV infections are asymptomatic and the only human virus isolates obtained from the initial 1995 outbreak were from two asymptomatic patients and these were only recovered after wider, retrospective sampling and surveillance of Torres Strait island residents was performed. Thus, some other form of active surveillance could potentially provide evidence as to whether the virus is still circulating in the Torres Strait.

When JEV first emerged in northern Australia it was initially feared that the virus would proliferate in mosquito–pig–bird cycles and become established on the mainland [50] similar to events involving establishment of WNV in bird-mosquito cycles in the United States [51]. Despite these predictions, viral activity appears to have remained restricted to the Torres Strait, with the occasional incursion onto Cape York Peninsula. There is no evidence to suggest that the virus has become established on the mainland, let alone reaching endemic status in any other areas of the country. Several ecological reasons for this apparent lack of establishment have been proposed and include: (a) competition between the endemic flaviviruses, MVEV and WNV_{KUN}, with JEV for susceptible vertebrate hosts; (b) host feeding patterns of *Cx. annulirostris* whereby they feed on hosts other than pigs, that cannot amplify JEV; and (c) different lineages of *Cx. annulirostris* which vary in their vector competence for the different genotypes of JEV [3]. Alternatively, the lack of detection on the mainland could represent the limited geographical area covered by the current sugar-based surveillance program. Whilst a vaccination program is in place for Torres Strait island residents, immunologically naïve populations exist on the mainland. Thus, it would be prudent to continue the current JEV surveillance program on Cape York Peninsula, and consider expanding its geographical scope with increased sensitivity to provide future early warning and enhanced public health prevention of disease.

The investigations presented in the current paper are, in effect, examples of One Health in action. Indeed, a One Health approach has been successfully used to understand JEV transmission and to provide tools to combat epidemics [5], and it has been suggested that the employment of One Health strategies, particularly those concerned with improving coordination and collaboration across different disciplines and jurisdictions, are essential to planning and initiating interventions to mitigate risk and in improving prevention and control of mosquito-borne arboviruses [52].

Author Contributions: Conceptualization, A.F.v.d.H., A.T.P., J.S.M., S.H.-M. and S.A.R.; Writing—Original Draft Preparation, A.F.v.d.H.; Writing—Review & Editing, A.F.v.d.H., A.T.P., J.S.M., S.H.-M. and S.A.R.

Funding: This research received no external funding.

Acknowledgments: The authors wish to thank Tim Kerlin, Keith Rickart and Jamie McMahon for information on recent JEV surveillance in Northern Australia. They also thank Frederick Moore for comments on the manuscript.

Conflicts of Interest: The authors declare no conflict of interest.

References

1. Campbell, G.L.; Hills, S.L.; Fischer, M.; Jacobson, J.A.; Hoke, C.H.; Hombach, J.M.; Marfin, A.A.; Solomon, T.; Tsai, T.F.; Tsu, V.D.; et al. Estimated global incidence of Japanese encephalitis: A systematic review. *Bull. World Health Organ.* **2011**, *89*, 766–774. [CrossRef]

2. Mackenzie, J.S.; Williams, D.T.; Smith, D.W. Japanese encephalitis virus: The geographic distribution, incidence, and spread of a virus with a propensity to emerge in new areas. *Perspect. Med. Virol.* **2006**, *16*, 201–268. [CrossRef]

3. Van den Hurk, A.F.; Ritchie, S.A.; Mackenzie, J.S. Ecology and geographical expansion of Japanese encephalitis virus. *Ann. Rev. Entomol.* **2009**, *54*, 17–35. [CrossRef] [PubMed]
4. Ricklin, M.E.; García-Nicolás, O.; Brechbühl, D.; Python, S.; Zumkehr, B.; Nougairede, A.; Charrel, R.N.; Posthaus, H.; Oevermann, A.; Summerfield, A. Vector-free transmission and persistence of Japanese encephalitis virus in pigs. *Nat. Commun.* **2016**, *7*, 10832. [CrossRef] [PubMed]
5. Impoinvil, D.E.; Baylis, M.; Solomon, T. Japanese encephalitis: On the One Health agenda. *Curr. Top. Microbiol. Immunol.* **2013**, *365*, 205–247. [CrossRef]
6. Fleming, K. Japanese encephalitis in an Australian soldier returned from Vietnam. *Med. J. Aust.* **1975**, *2*, 19–23. [PubMed]
7. Hanson, J.P.; Taylor, C.T.; Richards, A.R.; Smith, I.L.; Boutlis, C.S. Japanese encephalitis acquired near Port Moresby: Implications for residents and travellers to Papua New Guinea. *Med. J. Aust.* **2004**, *181*, 282.
8. Macdonald, W.B.G.; Tink, A.R.; Ouvrier, R.A.; Menser, M.A.; de Silva, L.M.; Naim, H.; Hawkes, R.A. Japanese encephalitis after a two-week holiday in Bali. *Med. J. Aust.* **1989**, *150*, 334–339.
9. Hanna, J.N.; Ritchie, S.A.; Phillips, D.A.; Shield, J.; Bailey, M.C.; Mackenzie, J.S.; Poidinger, M.; McCall, B.J.; Mills, P.J. An outbreak of Japanese encephalitis in the Torres Strait, Australia, 1995. *Med. J. Aust.* **1996**, *165*, 256–260.
10. Ritchie, S.A.; Phillips, D.; Broom, A.; Mackenzie, J.; Poidinger, M.; van den Hurk, A. Isolation of Japanese encephalitis virus from *Culex annulirostris* in Australia. *Am. J. Trop. Med. Hyg.* **1997**, *56*, 80–84. [CrossRef]
11. Ritchie, S.A.; van den Hurk, A.F.; Shield, J. The 1995 Japanese encephalitis outbreak: Why Badu? *Arbovirus Res. Aust.* **1997**, *7*, 224–227.
12. Hanna, J.; Barnett, D.; Ewald, D. Vaccination against Japanese encephalitis in the Torres Strait. *Comm. Dis. Intell.* **1996**, *19*, 447.
13. Shield, J.; Hanna, J.; Phillips, D. Reappearance of the Japanese encephalitis virus in the Torres Strait, 1996. *Comm. Dis. Intell.* **1996**, *20*, 191.
14. Johansen, C.A.; van den Hurk, A.F.; Ritchie, S.A.; Zborowski, P.; Paru, R.; Bockari, M.J.; Drew, A.C.; Khromykh, T.I.; Mackenzie, J.S. Isolation of Japanese encephalitis virus from mosquitoes (Diptera: Culicidae) collected in the Western Province of Papua New Guinea, 1997–1998. *Am. J. Trop. Med. Hyg.* **2000**, *62*, 631–638. [CrossRef] [PubMed]
15. Johansen, C.; Ritchie, S.; Hurk, A.v.d.; Bockarie, M.; Hanna, J.; Phillips, D.; Melrose, W.; Poidinger, M.; Scherret, J.; Hall, R.; et al. The Search for Japanese encephalitis virus in the Western Province of Papua New Guinea, 1996. *Arbovirus Res. Aust.* **1997**, *7*, 131–136.
16. Ritchie, S.A.; Rochester, W. Wind-blown mosquitoes and introduction of Japanese encephalitis into Australia. *Emerg. Infect. Dis.* **2001**, *7*, 900–903. [CrossRef]
17. Hanna, J.N.; Ritchie, S.A.; Phillips, D.A.; Lee, J.M.; Hills, S.; van den Hurk, A.F.; Pyke, A.; Johansen, C.A.; Mackenzie, J.S. Japanese encephalitis in north Queensland, Australia, 1998. *Med. J. Aust.* **1999**, *170*, 533–536. [CrossRef]
18. Johansen, C.A.; van den Hurk, A.F.; Pyke, A.T.; Zborowski, P.; Phillips, D.A.; Mackenzie, J.S.; Ritchie, J.S. Entomological Investigations of an outbreak of Japanese encephalaitis virus in the Torres Strait, Australia, in 1998. *J. Med. Entomol.* **2001**, *38*, 581–588. [CrossRef]
19. Van den Hurk, A.F.; Johansen, C.A.; Zborowski, P.; Phillips, D.A.; Pyke, A.T.; Mackenzie, J.S.; Ritchie, S.A. Flaviviruses isolated from mosquitoes collected during the first outbreak of Japanese encephalitis virus on Cape York Peninsula, Australia. *Am. J. Trop. Med. Hyg.* **2001**, *64*, 125–130. [CrossRef]
20. Barr, J. Drought Assessment: The 1997-98 El Nino Drought in Papua New Guinea and the Solomon Islands. *Aust. J. Emerg. Manag.* **1999**, *14*, 31–37.
21. Van den Hurk, A.F.; Nisbet, D.J.; Johansen, C.A.; Foley, P.N.; Ritchie, S.A.; Mackenzie, J.S. Japanese encephalitis on Badu Island, Australia: The first isolation of Japanese encephalitis virus from *Culex gelidus* in the Australasian region and the role of mosquito host-feeding patterns in virus transmission cycles. *Trans. Royal. Soc. Trop. Med. Hyg.* **2001**, *95*, 595–600. [CrossRef]
22. Johansen, C.A.; Nisbet, D.J.; Foley, P.N.; van den Hurk, A.F.; Hall, R.A.; Mackenzie, J.S.; Ritchie, S.A. Flavivirus isolations from mosquitoes collected from Saibai Island in the Torres Strait, Australia, during an incursion of Japanese encephalitis virus. *Med. Vet. Entomol.* **2004**, *18*, 281–287. [CrossRef]

23. Pyke, A.T.; Williams, D.T.; Nisbet, D.J.; van den Hurk, A.F.; Taylor, C.T.; Johansen, C.A.; Macdonald, J.; Hall, R.A.; Simmons, R.J.; Mason, R.J.V.; et al. The appearance of a second genotype of Japanese encephalitis virus in the Australasian region. *Am. J. Trop. Med. Hyg.* **2001**, *65*, 747–753. [CrossRef] [PubMed]

24. Ritchie, S.A.; van den Hurk, A.F.; Zborowski, P.; Kerlin, T.J.; Banks, D.; Walker, J.A.; Lee, J.M.; Montgomery, B.L.; Smith, G.A.; Pyke, A.T.; et al. Operational trials of remote mosquito trap systems for Japanese encephalitis virus surveillance in the Torres Strait, Australia. *Vector Borne Zoonotic Dis.* **2007**, *7*, 497–506. [CrossRef] [PubMed]

25. Van den Hurk, A.F.; Montgomery, B.L.; Northill, J.A.; Smith, I.L.; Zborowski, P.; Ritchie, S.A.; Mackenzie, J.S.; Smith, G.A. The first isolation of Japanese encephalitis virus from mosquitoes collected from mainland Australia. *Am. J. Trop. Med. Hyg.* **2006**, *75*, 21–25. [CrossRef]

26. Johnson, B.J.; Kerlin, T.; Hall-Mendelin, S.; van den Hurk, A.F.; Cortis, G.; Doggett, S.L.; Toi, C.; Fall, K.; McMahon, J.L.; Townsend, M.; et al. Development and field evaluation of the sentinel mosquito arbovirus capture kit (SMACK). *Parasit. Vectors* **2015**, *8*, 509. [CrossRef]

27. Boyle, D.B.; Dickerman, R.W.; Marshall, I.D. Primary viraemia responses of herons to experimental infection with Murray Valley encephalitis, Kunjin and Japanese encephalitis viruses. *Aust. J. Exp. Biol. Med. Sci.* **1983**, *61*, 655–664. [CrossRef]

28. Mackenzie, J.S.; Johansen, C.A.; Ritchie, S.A.; van den Hurk, A.F.; Hall, R.A. The emergence and spread of Japanese encephalitis virus in Australasia. *Curr. Top. Microbiol. Immunol.* **2002**, *267*, 49–73. [CrossRef]

29. Van den Hurk, A.F.; Smith, C.S.; Field, H.E.; Smith, I.L.; Northill, J.A.; Taylor, C.T.; Jansen, C.C.; Smith, G.A.; Mackenzie, J.S. Transmission of Japanese encephalitis virus from the black flying fox, *Pteropus alecto*, to *Culex annulirostris* mosquitoes, despite the absence of detectable viremia. *Am. J. Trop. Med. Hyg.* **2009**, *81*, 457–462. [CrossRef]

30. Williams, D.T.; Daniels, P.W.; Lunt, R.A.; Wang, L.-F.; Newberry, K.M.; Mackenzie, J.S. Experimental infections of pigs with Japanese encephalitis virus and closely related Australian flaviviruses. *Am. J. Trop. Med. Hyg.* **2001**, *65*, 379–387. [CrossRef]

31. Van den Hurk, A.F.; Jansen, C.C. Arboviruses of Oceania. In *Neglected Tropical Diseases—Oceania*; Loukas, A., Ed.; Springer Nature: Basel, Switzerland, 2016; pp. 193–235. [CrossRef]

32. Van den Hurk, A.F.; Nisbet, D.J.; Hall, R.A.; Kay, B.H.; Mackenzie, J.S.; Ritchie, S.A. Vector competence of Australian mosquitoes (Diptera: Culicidae) for Japanese encephalitis virus. *J. Med. Entomol.* **2003**, *40*, 82–90. [CrossRef] [PubMed]

33. Hemmerter, S.; Slapeta, J.; van den Hurk, A.F.; Cooper, R.D.; Whelan, P.I.; Russell, R.C.; Johansen, C.A.; Beebe, N.W. A curious coincidence: Mosquito biodiversity and the limits of the Japanese encephalitis virus in Australasia. *BMC Evol. Biol.* **2007**, *7*, 100. [CrossRef] [PubMed]

34. Johnson, P.H.; Hall-Mendelin, S.; Whelan, P.I.; Frances, S.P.; Jansen, C.C.; Mackenzie, D.O.; Northill, J.A.; van den Hurk, A.F. Vector competence of Australian *Culex gelidus* Theobald (Diptera: Culicidae) for endemic and exotic arboviruses. *Aust. J. Entomol.* **2009**, *48*, 234–240. [CrossRef]

35. Chapman, H.F.; Kay, B.H.; Ritchie, S.A.; van den Hurk, A.F.; Hughes, J.M. Definition of species in the *Culex sitiens* subgroup (Diptera: Culicidae) from Papua New Guinea and Australia. *J. Med. Entomol.* **2000**, *37*, 736–742. [CrossRef] [PubMed]

36. Hall-Mendelin, S.; Jansen, C.C.; Cheah, W.Y.; Montgomery, B.L.; Hall, R.A.; Ritchie, S.A.; van den Hurk, A.F. *Culex annulirostris* (Diptera: Culicidae) host feeding patterns and Japanese encephalitis virus ecology in northern Australia. *J. Med. Entomol.* **2012**, *49*, 371–377. [CrossRef] [PubMed]

37. Van den Hurk, A.F.; Johansen, C.A.; Zborowski, P.; Paru, R.; Foley, P.N.; Beebe, N.W.; Mackenzie, J.S.; Ritchie, S.A. Mosquito host-feeding patterns and implications for Japanese encephalitis virus transmission in northern Australia and Papua New Guinea. *Med. Vet. Entomol.* **2003**, *17*, 403–411. [CrossRef]

38. Van den Hurk, A.F.; Smith, I.L.; Smith, G.A. Development and evaluation of real-time polymerase chain reaction assays to identify mosquito (Diptera: Culicidae) blood meals originating from native Australian mammals. *J. Med. Entomol.* **2007**, *44*, 85–92. [CrossRef]

39. Van den Hurk, A.F.; Ritchie, S.A.; Johansen, C.A.; Mackenzie, J.S.; Smith, G.A. Domestic pigs and Japanese encephalitis virus infection, Australia. *Emerg. Infect. Dis.* **2008**, *14*, 1736–1738. [CrossRef]

40. Bryan, J.H.; O'Donnell, M.S.; Berry, G.; Carvan, T. Dispersal of adult female *Culex annulirostris* in Griffith, New South Wales, Australia: A further study. *J. Am. Mosq. Control. Assoc.* **1992**, *8*, 398–403.

41. Van den Hurk, A.F.; Johnson, P.H.; Hall-Mendelin, S.; Northill, J.A.; Simmons, R.J.; Jansen, C.C.; Frances, S.P.; Smith, G.A.; Ritchie, S.A. Expectoration of flaviviruses during sugar feeding by mosquitoes (Diptera: Culicidae). *J. Med. Entomol.* **2007**, *44*, 845–850. [CrossRef]

42. Hall-Mendelin, S.; Ritchie, S.A.; Johansen, C.A.; Zborowski, P.; Cortis, G.; Dandridge, S.; Hall, R.A.; van den Hurk, A.F. Exploiting mosquito sugar feeding to detect mosquito-borne pathogens. *Proc. Natl. Acad. Sci. USA* **2010**, *107*, 11255–11259. [CrossRef] [PubMed]

43. Ritchie, S.A.; Cortis, G.; Paton, C.; Townsend, M.; Shroyer, D.; Zborowski, P.; Hall-Mendelin, S.; van den Hurk, A.F. A simple non-powered passive trap for the collection of mosquitoes for arbovirus surveillance. *J. Med. Entomol.* **2013**, *50*, 185–194. [CrossRef] [PubMed]

44. Huang, B.; Firth, C.; Watterson, D.; Allcock, R.; Colmant, A.M.; Hobson-Peters, J.; Kirkland, P.; Hewitson, G.; McMahon, J.; Hall-Mendelin, S.; et al. Genetic characterization of archived Bunyaviruses and their potential for emergence in Australia. *Emerg. Infect. Dis.* **2016**, *22*, 833–840. [CrossRef] [PubMed]

45. Van den Hurk, A.F.; Hall-Mendelin, S.; Townsend, M.; Kurucz, N.; Edwards, J.; Ehlers, G.; Rodwell, C.; Moore, F.A.; McMahon, J.L.; Northill, J.A.; et al. Applications of a sugar-based surveillance system to track arboviruses in wild mosquito populations. *Vector Borne Zoonotic Dis.* **2014**, *14*, 66–73. [CrossRef] [PubMed]

46. Ramirez, A.L.; Hall-Mendelin, S.; Doggett, S.L.; Hewitson, G.R.; McMahon, J.L.; Ritchie, S.A.; van den Hurk, A.F. Mosquito excreta: A sample type with many potential applications for the investigation of Ross River virus and West Nile virus ecology. *PLoS Negl. Trop. Dis.* **2018**, *12*, e0006771. [CrossRef] [PubMed]

47. Fontaine, A.; Jiolle, D.; Moltini-Conclois, I.; Lequime, S.; Lambrechts, L. Excretion of dengue virus RNA by *Aedes aegypti* allows non-destructive monitoring of viral dissemination in individual mosquitoes. *Sci. Rep.* **2016**, *6*, 24885. [CrossRef]

48. Australian Technical Advisory Group on Immunisation. *Australian Immunisation Handbook*; Australian Government Department of Health: Canberra, Australia, 2018. Available online: https://immunisationhandbook.health.gov.au/ (accessed on 18 February 2019).

49. Australian Government Department of Health. Japanese Encephalitis Virus Infection Case Definition—V1.1. Available online: http://www.health.gov.au/internet/main/publishing.nsf/Content/cda-surveil-nndss-casedefs-cd_je.htm (accessed on 18 February 2019).

50. Mackenzie, J.S.; Broom, A.K.; Hall, R.A.; Johansen, C.A.; Lindsay, M.D.; Phillips, D.A.; Ritchie, S.A.; Russell, R.C.; Smith, D.W. Arboviruses in the Australian region, 1990 to 1998. *Comm. Dis. Intell.* **1998**, *22*, 93–100.

51. Mackenzie, J.S.; Gubler, D.J.; Petersen, L.R. Emerging flaviviruses: The spread and resurgence of Japanese encephalitis, West Nile and dengue viruses. *Nature Med.* **2004**, *10*, S98–S109. [CrossRef]

52. Mackenzie, J.S.; Lindsay, M.D.A.; Smith, D.W.; Imrie, A. The ecology and epidemiology of Ross River and Murray Valley encephalitis viruses in Western Australia: Examples of One Health in action. *Trans. R. Soc. Trop. Med. Hyg.* **2017**, *111*, 248–254. [CrossRef]

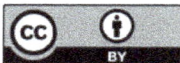

Tropical Medicine and Infectious Disease

MDPI

Review

One Health—Its Importance in Helping to Better Control Antimicrobial Resistance

Peter J. Collignon [1,2,*] and Scott A. McEwen [3]

[1] Infectious Diseases and Microbiology, Canberra Hospital, Garran, ACT 2605, Australia
[2] Medical School, Australian National University, Acton ACT 2601, Australia
[3] Department of Population Medicine, University of Guelph, Guelph N1G 2W1, Canada; smcewen@uoguelph.ca
* Correspondence: peter.collignon@act.gov.au

Received: 27 December 2018; Accepted: 23 January 2019; Published: 29 January 2019

Abstract: Approaching any issue from a One Health perspective necessitates looking at the interactions of people, domestic animals, wildlife, plants, and our environment. For antimicrobial resistance this includes antimicrobial use (and abuse) in the human, animal and environmental sectors. More importantly, the spread of resistant bacteria and resistance determinants within and between these sectors and globally must be addressed. Better managing this problem includes taking steps to preserve the continued effectiveness of existing antimicrobials such as trying to eliminate their inappropriate use, particularly where they are used in high volumes. Examples are the mass medication of animals with critically important antimicrobials for humans, such as third generation cephalosporins and fluoroquinolones, and the long term, in-feed use of antimicrobials, such colistin, tetracyclines and macrolides, for growth promotion. In people it is essential to better prevent infections, reduce over-prescribing and over-use of antimicrobials and stop resistant bacteria from spreading by improving hygiene and infection control, drinking water and sanitation. Pollution from inadequate treatment of industrial, residential and farm waste is expanding the resistome in the environment. Numerous countries and several international agencies have now included a One Health Approach within their action plans to address antimicrobial resistance. Necessary actions include improvements in antimicrobial use, better regulation and policy, as well as improved surveillance, stewardship, infection control, sanitation, animal husbandry, and finding alternatives to antimicrobials.

Keywords: One Health; antibiotics; antimicrobials; antimicrobial resistance; environment; water; infrastructure

1. Introduction

Antimicrobial resistance is a global public health problem [1,2]. Most bacteria that cause serious infections and could once be successfully treated with several different antibiotic classes, have now acquired resistance—often to many antibiotics. In some regions the increased resistance has been so extensive that resistance is present in some bacteria to nearly all of these drugs [2–4]. The threat is most acute for antibacterial antimicrobials (antibiotics—the focus of this paper) but also threatens antifungals, antiparastics and antivirals [5].

Antimicrobial overuse is occurring in multiple sectors (human, animal, agriculture) [3,6]. Microorganisms faced with antimicrobial selection pressure enhance their fitness by acquiring and expressing resistance genes, then sharing them with other bacteria and by other mechanisms, for example gene overexpression and silencing, phase variation. When bacteria are resistant they also present in much larger numbers when exposed to antimicrobials, whether in an individual, in a location and in the environment. Additionally important in driving the deteriorating resistance problem are factors that promote the spread of resistant bacteria (or "contagion") [7]. This spread involves not only bacteria themselves but the resistance genes they carry and that can be acquired by other bacteria [8]. Factors that facilitate "contagion" include poverty, poor housing, poor infection control, poor water supplies, poor sanitation, run off of waste from intensive agriculture, environmental contamination and geographical movement of infected humans and animals [9–11].

Wherever antimicrobials are used, there are often already large reservoirs of resistant bacteria and resistance genes. These include people and their local environments (both in hospitals and in the community), as well as animals, farms and aquaculture environments. Large reservoirs of resistance and residual antimicrobials occur in water, soil, wildlife and many other ecological niches, not only due to pollution by sewage, pharmaceutical industry waste and manure runoff from farms [10,12,13], but often resistant bacteria and resistance genes have already been there for millennia [14,15].

Most bacteria and their genes can move relatively easily within and between humans, animals and the environment. Microbial adaptations to antimicrobial use and other selection pressures within any one sector are reflected in other sectors [8,16]. Similarly, actions (or inactions) to contain antimicrobial resistance in one sector affect other sectors [17,18]. Antimicrobial resistance is an ecological problem that is characterized by complex interactions involving diverse microbial populations affecting the health of humans, animals and the environment. It makes sense to address the resistance problem by taking this complexity and ecological nature into account using a coordinated, multi-sectoral approach, such as One Health [5,19–23].

One Health is defined by WHO [24] and others [25] as a concept and approach to "designing and implementing programs, policies, legislation and research in which multiple sectors communicate and work together to achieve better public health outcomes. The areas of work in which a One Health approach is particularly relevant include food safety, the control of zoonoses and combatting antibiotic resistance" [24]. It needs to involve the "collaborative effort of multiple health science professions, together with their related disciplines and institutions—working locally, nationally, and globally—to attain optimal health for people, domestic animals, wildlife, plants, and our environment" [25]. The origins of One Health are centuries old and are based on the mutual inter-dependence of people and animals and a recognition that they share not only the same environment, but also many infectious diseases [23]. Our current concept of One Health however goes much further. It also embraces the health of the environment.

2. Use of Antimicrobials in Humans, Animals and Plants

The vast majority of antimicrobial classes are used both in humans and animals (including aquaculture; both farmed fish and shellfish). Only few antimicrobial classes are reserved exclusively for humans (e.g., carbapenems). There are also few classes limited to veterinary use (e.g., flavophospholipols, ionophores); mainly because of toxicity to humans [26–30].

Insects (e.g., bees) and some plants are frequently treated with antimicrobials. Tetracyclines, streptomycin and some other antimicrobials are used for treatment and prophylaxis of bacterial infections of fruit, such as apples and pears (e.g., "fire blight" caused by *Erwinia amylovora*) [31,32]. Antifungals, especially azoles, are used in huge quantities and applied to broad acre crops such as wheat [33].

There are marked differences in the ways antimicrobials are used in human compared to non-human sectors. In people, antimicrobials are mostly used for treatment of clinical infections in individual patients, with some limited prophylactic use in individuals (e.g., post-surgery) or occasionally in groups (e.g., prevention of meningococcal disease). Antimicrobial uses in companion animals (e.g., dogs, cats, pet birds, horses) are broadly similar to those in humans, with antimicrobials mostly administered on an individual basis to treat infection, and occasionally for prophylaxis, such as post-surgery [34,35].

In the food-producing animal sector, antimicrobials are also used therapeutically to treat individual clinically sick animals (e.g., dairy cows with mastitis) [26]. However, in intensive farming and aquaculture, for reasons of practicality and efficiency, antimicrobials are often administered through feed or water to entire groups (e.g., pens of pigs, flocks of broilers), either for prophylaxis (to healthy animals at risk of infection) or metaphylaxis (to healthy animals in the same group as diseased animals) [36]. Some have even succeeded in having this group level administration defined (and we believe inappropriately) in the animal health sector as "therapeutic" use. Growth promotion, prophylaxis and metaphylaxis account for by far the largest volumes of antimicrobials used in the food-producing animal sector [26,27,37].

Growth Promotion Use

Using antimicrobials for growth promotion is highly controversial because instead of treating sick animals they are administered to healthy animals, usually for prolonged periods of time, and often at sub-therapeutic doses in order to improve production. These conditions favor selection and spread of resistant bacteria within animals and to humans through food or other environmental pathways [38,39]. The period of exposure with growth promotion is usually greater than two weeks and often almost the entire life of an animal, for example in chicken for 36 days or more.

Based on studies, mostly conducted decades ago, the purported production benefits of antimicrobial growth promoters range widely (1–10%). Surveillance and animal production data however now suggests that benefits in animals reared in good conditions are probably quite small and may be non-existent. Many large poultry corporations are now marketing chicken raised without antimicrobials administered at hatchery or farm levels [40]. Expressed concerns are that antimicrobial growth promoters are used to compensate for poor hygiene and housing, and as replacement for proper animal health management [18,41,42]. For these reasons, the World Health Organization (WHO) advocates the termination of antimicrobial use for growth promotion [5,41]. This practice has now been banned in Europe and elsewhere and is being phased out in some other countries [43–45]. However there are still many countries where they continue to be used [46], including drugs categorized by WHO as critically important to humans, for example colistin, fluoroquinolones and macrolides [47].

Comprehensive global quantitative data on use of antimicrobial agents in humans, animals and plants is generally lacking. Table 1 shows the varying levels of antibiotic usage in people around the world, associated resistance levels, plus some social and infrastructure parameters—the latter of which can facilitate the spread of resistant bacteria (e.g., poor sanitation). Figure 1 shows antibiotic use in different regions globally in people and the lack of correlation with increased resistance levels in bacteria and human antibiotic usage. These data strongly suggest that there are other very important factors influencing antimicrobial resistance over and above simply antibiotic usage.

Table 1. Levels of antibiotic usage in people, resistance levels and other parameters globally. (All data taken from reference 7).

Country	Antibiotic Usage (Standard units per 1000 pop - CCDEP)	E. coli % Resistance 3rd gen ceph (WHO)	E. coli % Resistance Fluoroquinolones (WHO)	Staphylococcus Aureus (MRSA Rates - WHO)	2015 Corruption Index	GNP per capita 2015 (Purchasing Power Parity in 2011 Dollars)	% with Adequate Sanitation 2015	Improved Water Source (% of Population with Access)
Algeria	15.4	17	2	44.8	36	$13,795	88	87.7
Argentina	6.2	5.1	7.8	54	32	$19,102	96	98.9
Australia	11	7.7	10.6	30	79	$43,631	100	100
Austria	7.2	9.1	22.3	7.4	76	$44,048	100	100
Bahrain		55	62	10	51	$43,754	99	100
Bangladesh	4.3	57.4	89	46	25	$3,137	61	86.2
Belgium	12.6	6	21.5	17.4	77	$41,826	100	100
Bhutan		19.4	35.5	10	65	$7,861	50	100
Bosnia and Herzegovina	7.5	1.5	7.8		38	$10,119	95	99.9
Brazil	5.9	30	40	29.5	38	$14,533	83	98.1
Brunei Darussalam		6.5	12		55	$73,605	100	100
Bulgaria	9.4	22.9	30.2	22.4	41	$17,000	86	99.6
Burkina Faso		36	52.8		38	$1,593	20	82.1
Burundi		7.2	16	13	21	$683	48	75.8
Cambodia		45	71.8		21	$3,278	42	73.4
Canada	7.2	8	26.9	21	83	$42,983	100	99.8
Central African Republic		30	53		24	$581	22	68.4
Chile	4.3	23.8		90	70	$22,197	99	99
China	3	51.9	55.1	38.3	70	$13,572	77	94.8
Colombia	2.9	11.7	59	7.2	37	$12,988	81	91.3
Croatia	10.6	6	14	13	51	$20,664	97	99.6
Cuba		42.9	56		47	$21,017	93	94.6
Cyprus		36.2	47.4	41.6	61	$30,363	100	100
Czech Republic	7.5	11.4	23.5	14.5	56	$30,381	99	100
Denmark	6.7	8.5	14.1	1.2	91	$45,484	100	100
Dominican Republic	2.4	33	49	30	33	$13,372	84	86.5
Ecuador	6.7	15.1	43.8	29	32	$10,777	85	86.9
Egypt	9.1	44.4	34.9	46	36	$10,250	95	99.2
Estonia	4.4		9.9	1.7	70	$27,345	97	99.6

Trop. Med. Infect. Dis. **2019**, *4*, 22

Table 1. *Cont.*

Country	Antibiotic Usage (Standard units per 1000 pop - CCDEP)	E. coli % Resistance 3rd gen ceph (WHO)	E. coli % Resistance Fluoroquinolones (WHO)	Staphylococcus Aureus (MRSA Rates - WHO)	2015 Corruption Index	GNP per capita 2015 (Purchasing Power Parity in 2011 Dollars)	% with Adequate Sanitation 2015	Improved Water Source (% of Population with Access)
Ethiopia		62	71	31.6	33	$1,530	28	55.4
Finland	7.2	5.1	10.8	2.8	90	$38,994	98	100
France	12.9	8.2	17.9	20.1	70	$37,775	99	100
Germany	7.1	8	23.7	16.2	81	$43,788	99	100
Greece	14.6	14.9	26.6	39.2	46	$24,095	99	100
Guatemala		39.8	41.8	52	28	$7,253	64	92.7
Honduras		36.7	43.1	30	31	$4,785	83	90.6
Hong Kong	7.5				75	$53,463	96	100
Hungary	7.3	15.1	31.2	26.2	51	$24,831	98	100
Iceland		6.2	14		79	$42,704	99	100
India	5	51.4	52.3	42.7	38	$5,733	40	94.1
Indonesia	3.6				36	$10,385	61	86.8
Iran		41	54	53	27	$16,507	90	96.2
Ireland	11.4	9	22.9	23.7	75	$61,378	91	97.9
Israel		2.6	17.9	46.7	61	$31,971	100	100
Italy	11.5	19.8	40.5	38.2	44	$34,220	100	100
Japan	5.3	16.6	34.3	53	75	$37,872	100	100
Jordan	6.3	22.5	14.5		53	$10,240	99	96.9
Kazakhstan	7.5				28	$23,522	98	93.5
Kenya		87.2	91.4	20	25	$2,901	30	63.1
Kuwait	6.3	20.1		32	49	$70,107	100	99
Latvia	5.2	15.9	16.8	9.9	55	$23,080	88	99.3
Lebanon	9.3	27.7	47	20	28	$13,089	81	99
Lesotho		2	14		44	$2,770	30	81.6
Lithuania	7.6	7	12.9	5.8	61	$26,971	92	96.6
Luxembourg	11	8.2	24.1	20.5	81	$93,900	98	100
Malaysia	4.3	17.4	23	17.3	50	$25,312	96	98.2
Malta		12.8	32	49.2	56	$32,720	100	100
Mexico	2.4	42.1	46.3	29.9	35	$16,490	85	96.1

Trop. Med. Infect. Dis. **2019**, *4*, 22

Table 1. *Cont.*

Country	Antibiotic Usage (Standard units per 1000 pop - CCDEP)	E. coli % Resistance 3rd gen ceph (WHO)	E. coli % Resistance Fluoroquinolones (WHO)	Staphylococcus Aureus (MRSA Rates - WHO)	2015 Corruption Index	GNP per capita 2015 (Purchasing Power Parity in 2011 Dollars)	% with Adequate Sanitation 2015	Improved Water Source (% of Population with Access)
Mongolia		64.1	64.7		39	$11,478	60	64.2
Morocco	6	4	23.3	19	36	$7,365	77	85.3
Myanmar		68	55	26	22	$4,931	80	80.5
Nepal		37.9	64.3	44.9	27	$2,312	46	90.7
Netherlands	4.1	5.7	14.3	1.4	87	$46,354	98	100
New Zealand	10.9	3	6.5	10.4	88	$35,159	100	100
Nicaragua		48.1	42.9		27	$4,884	68	86.9
Nigeria		6.7	36.5	47.1	26	$5,639	29	67.6
Norway	5.9	3.6	9	0.3	87	$63,650	98	100
Pakistan	7.1	36.2	35.3	37.6	30	$4,706	64	91.3
Panama		9.2	23.3	21.1	39	$20,885	75	94.4
Papua New Guinea			13.3	43.9	25	$2,723	19	40
Paraguay	3.4	1.4	22.1	27	27	$8,639	89	96.6
Peru		44.1	62.8	65.9	36	$11,768	76	86.3
Philippines	2.2	26.7	40.9	54.9	35	$6,938	74	91.5
Poland	9.3	11.7	27.3	24.3	62	$25,323	97	98.3
Portugal	9.3	11.3	27.2	54.6	63	$26,549	100	100
Puerto Rico	9.1						99	
Republic of Moldova		28	15.3	50.3	33	$4,742	76	88.4
Russian Federation	6.2	18	25.7	29.3	29	$24,124	72	96.9
Rwanda		21.4			54	$1,655	62	75.5
Serbia	10.6	21.3	16	44.5	40	$13,278	96	99.3
Singapore	5.7	20	37.8		85	$80,192	100	100
Slovakia	9.2	31	41.9	25.9	51	$28,254	99	100
Slovenia	6.3	8.8	20.7	7.1	60	$29,097	99	99.6
South Africa	8.7	8.2	16.1	52	44	$12,393	66	92.8
South Korea	10.9	24.4	40.9	65.3	56	$34,387	100	97.6
Spain	14.3	12	34.5	22.5	55	$32,219	100	100
Sri Lanka	3.9	58.9	58.8		37	$11,048	95	95.6

Table 1. *Cont.*

Country	Antibiotic Usage (Standard units per 1000 pop - CCDEP)	E. coli % Resistance 3rd gen ceph (WHO)	E. coli % Resistance Fluoroquinolones (WHO)	Staphylococcus Aureus (MRSA Rates - WHO)	2015 Corruption Index	GNP per capita 2015 (Purchasing Power Parity in 2011 Dollars)	% with Adequate Sanitation 2015	Improved Water Source (% of Population with Access)
Sudan		49.5	56.8		12	$4,121	24	58.5
Saudi Arabia	11.1	15.9	40.9	41.9	52	$50,284	100	97
Sweden	4.8	3	7.9	0.8	89	$45,488	99	100
Switzerland	5.2	8.2	20.2	10.2	86	$56,517	100	100
Syrian Arab Republic		49.8			18	$-	96	90.1
Taiwan	8.7				62			
Thailand	7	37.9	52.5	22.4	38	$15,347	93	97.8
Tunisia	18	20.6	9.4	55.8	38	$10,770	92	97.7
Turkey	18.5	43.3	46.3	31.5	42	$19,460	95	100
United Arab Emirates	10.5	23	32.5	33.4	70	$65,717	98	99.7
United Kingdom	9	9.6	17.5	13.6	81	$38,509	99	100
United States of America	10.3	14.6	33.3	51.3	76	$52,704	100	99.2
Uruguay	6.6	0	15	40	74	$19,952	96	99.6
Venezuela	8.1	12.5	37.2	31	17	$16,769	94	93.1
Vietnam	9.4		0.2		31	$5,667	78	96.4
Zambia		37.4	50.5	32	38	$3,602	44	64.6

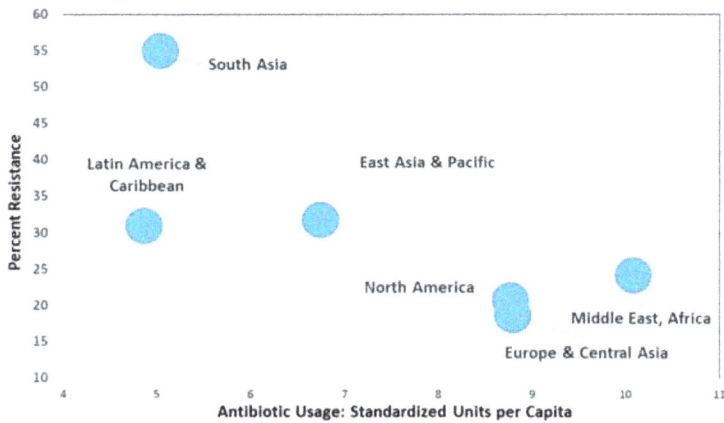

Figure 1. Global aggregated regions: antimicrobial resistance *E. coli* to third generation cephalosporins and fluoroquinolones versus antibiotic usage.

Aggregating countries into regional groupings shows a pattern where there is an inverse aggregate relationship between antimicrobial resistance and usage. These data help confirm that there are other very important factors influencing antimicrobial resistance over and above simply antibiotic usage. (Figures assembled from data taken from reference 7)

The World Organization for Animal Health has developed a global database on the use of antimicrobial agents in animals [46]. Figure 2 shows reported quantities of antimicrobials used in animals in 2014, summarized by OIE Region and expressed as total quantities (tons) and adjusted for animal biomass. Additionally, included is the per cent of countries authorizing the use of antimicrobials for growth promotion. Tetracyclines accounted for the largest proportion of overall antimicrobial use globally (37.1% of total), followed by polypeptides (15.7%), penicillins (9.8%), macrolides (8.9%) and aminoglycosides (7.8%) [46].

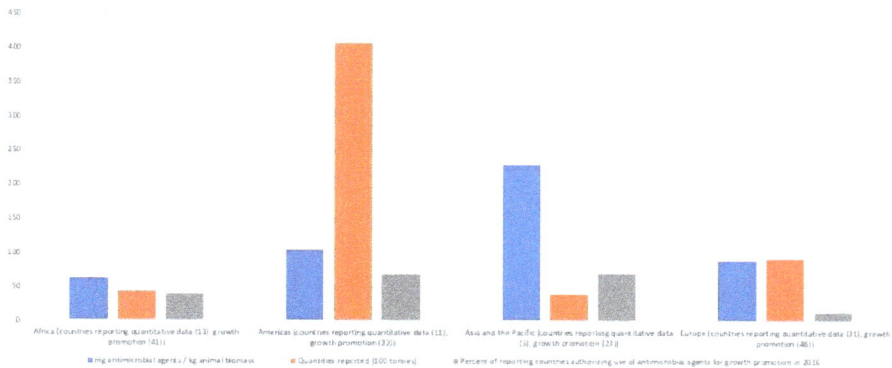

Figure 2. Reported use of antimicrobial agents in animals in 2014 by World Organisation for Animal Health (OIE) Region (adapted from [46]).

3. One Health Antimicrobial Resistance Case Studies

The following examples illustrate antimicrobial resistance problems that arise when the same classes of antimicrobials are used in humans and animals, and the challenges that arise from competing interests and imbalances of risk and benefit in various sectors.

3.1. Third Generation Cephalosporins

Third generation cephalosporins are broad spectrum beta-lactam antimicrobials that are widely used in humans and animals. In people, cefotaxime, ceftriaxone and several other members of the class are used for a wide variety of frequently serious infections, particularly in hospital settings, for example bloodstream infections due to *Escherichia coli* and other bacteria, but also in community settings, for example *Neisseria gonorrhea* [47]. Third generation cephalosporins are classified as "critically important" for human health [47].

Ceftiofur is the principal third generation cephalosporin for veterinary use; others include cefpodoxime, cefoperazone and cefovecin. Ceftiofur is injected and used in animals as therapy to treat pneumonia, arthritis, septicemia and other conditions [48,49]. However ceftiofur is also used in mass therapy (metaphylaxis or prophylaxis), either under an approved label claim (e.g., injection of feedlot cattle for control of bovine respiratory disease), or off-label (e.g., injection of hatching eggs or day-old chicks for prevention of *E. coli* infections). Factors that encourage overuse of ceftiofur are its broad spectrum activity, zero withdrawal time for milk from dairy animals (due to its high maximum residual level; MRL), and availability of a long-acting preparation [48,49].

In Europe, approximately 14 tons of third and fourth generation cephalosporins were used in 2014 for use in animals [28]. Similar volumes are used in the US [50]. In many countries, cephalosporins are commonly used in humans but with wide variations. Overall, 101 tons of third generation cephalosporins were used in people Europe in 2012 [29] and in the US, approximately 82 tons in 2011 [51].

Resistance to the third generation cephalosporins is mainly mediated by extended-spectrum beta-lactamases (ESBLs) and AmpC beta-lactamases [47]. ESBL genes are highly mobile and transmitted on plasmids, transposons and other genetic elements. AmpC beta-lactamases were originally reported to be chromosomal but have also been identified on plasmids and to have spread horizontally among *Enterobacteriaceae* [47]. Unfortunately, in many countries resistance to third generation cephalosporins is now common among *E. coli* and *K. pneumonia* [52,53]. Resistance genes are frequently co-located with genes encoding resistance to other classes of antimicrobials, including tetracyclines, aminoglycosides and sulfonamides. As a consequence, the use of other antimicrobials in animals, for example tetracyclines administered in feed, can select for ESBL strains of bacteria [54].

Ceftiofur can be administered to eggs or day-old chicks in hatcheries, using automated equipment that injects small quantities of the drug into the many thousands of hatching eggs or chicks intended for treated flocks as prophylaxis against *E. coli* infections [55,56]. This practice selected for cephalosporin resistance in *Salmonella* Heidelberg, an important cause of human illness and associated with consumption of poultry products [57]. Surveillance detected a high degree of time-related correlations in trends of resistance to ceftiofur (and ceftriaxone, a drug of choice for treatment of severe cases of salmonellosis in children and pregnant women) among *Salmonella* Heidelberg from clinical infections in humans, from poultry samples collected at retail, and in *E. coli* from retail poultry samples [55]. Voluntary termination of ceftiofur use in hatcheries in Quebec was followed by a precipitous drop in the prevalence of resistance to ceftiofur. Subsequent re-introduction of its use, was followed by a return to higher prevalence of resistance [56]. In recognition of the resultant human health risks, in 2014, the Canadian poultry industry placed a voluntary ban on the use of ceftiofur and other critically important antimicrobials for disease prophylaxis [58].

In Japan, voluntary withdrawal of the off-label use of ceftiofur in hatcheries in 2012 was also followed by a significant decrease in broad-spectrum cephalosporin resistance in *E. coli* from broilers [59]. Some other countries (e.g., Denmark and Australia) have also placed voluntary restrictions in its use [60]. The label claim for day-old injection of poultry flocks was withdrawn in Europe, while some countries banned off-label use of third generation cephalosporins (e.g., U.S.) [48,61], and in other countries there is a requirement that use is restricted to situations where no other effective approved drugs are available for treatment [62].

3.2. Colistin

Colistin is in the polymyxin class of antimicrobials, and has been used in both people and animals for over 50 years [63]. Polymyxins, when administered systemically, frequently cause nephrotoxicity and neurotoxicity in people [64]. Thus, until recently its use was mainly limited to topical use and the treatment of infections in cystic fibrosis patients by inhalation (with a colistimethate sodium).

Colistin however is now used much more frequently, as a drug of last resort by injection, for treatment of multi-resistant gram-negative infections including carbapenem-resistant *Pseudomonas aeruginosa* and *E. coli* [65–67]. Where approved for use in food animals (e.g., Brazil, Europe, China), most colistin is administered orally to groups of pigs, poultry and in some cases calves, for treatment and prophylaxis of diarrhea due to gram-negative infections or for growth promotion [63,67,68]. In countries where data are available, the quantities consumed for animal production vastly exceed those used in humans and is very variable between countries [69]. In 2013 total animal consumption in Europe was 495 tons; 99.7% in oral form (e.g., for oral solution, medicated feed premix and oral powder) [63]. In China, the world's largest producer of pigs and poultry, an estimated 12,000 tons of colistin was used in food animals [68].

Until recently, limited data on colistin resistance were available, partly because of technical difficulties in phenotypic susceptibility testing [63,70]. In Europe in 2016, resistance was found in 1.9% of indicator *E. coli* from broilers, 3.9% from broiler meat, 6.1% from turkeys and 10.1% from turkey meat [71]. Colistin resistance was thought limited to chromosomal mutation and was essentially non-transferable [63], however in 2015 the transferable plasmid-mediated colistin resistance gene, mcr-1, was found in *E. coli* isolates obtained from animals, food and human bloodstream infections from China [68]. Spread of the gene by conjugation has been shown in *Klebsiella pneumoniae*, *Enterobacter aerogenes*, *Enterobacter spp.* and *P. aeruginosa* [68]. Retrospective analyses have demonstrated the mcr-1 gene in several bacterial species isolated from humans, animals and environmental samples in numerous countries [72–76], and the gene was found in about 5% of healthy travelers [77]. The earliest identification of the gene thus far was in *E. coli* from poultry collected in the 1980s in China [78]. The mcr-1 gene has also been detected in isolates obtained from wildlife and surface water samples, demonstrating environmental contamination [79]. Recently, other plasmid-mediated colistin resistance genes has been reported for example mcr-2 in *E. coli* from pigs in Belgium [80].

Colistin illustrates some important One Health dimensions of antimicrobial resistance that differ from those of third generation cephalosporins. The toxicity with systemic use and the availability of other safer and more effective antimicrobials, meant for many years colistin was mainly used topically in people. However with the emergence of multi-drug resistance in many Gram-negative bacteria, there has been increasing need for this drug to systemically treat severe, life-threatening infections in humans in many countries. The colistin case demonstrates (once again) that using large quantities antimicrobials for group treatments or growth promotion in animals can lead to significant antimicrobial resistance problems for human health, even if the drug class is initially believed to be of lesser importance, because the relative importance of antimicrobials to human health can change. This is the same problem that arose from using avoparcin as a growth promoter until it was banned; it selected for resistance to another glycopeptide, vancomycin, which is used for the treatment of life-threatening MRSA (methicillin resistant *Staphylococcus aureus*) and for treating serious enterococcal infections (the latter especially in penicillin allergic patients) [81,82].

4. Risks to Public Health and Animal Health

Antimicrobial resistance is harmful to health because it reduces the effectiveness of antimicrobial therapy and tends to increase the severity, incidence and costs of infection [3,83]. There is now considerable evidence that antimicrobial use in animals is an important contributor to antimicrobial resistance among some pathogens of humans, in particular, common enteric pathogens such as *Salmonella spp.*, *Campylobacter spp.*, *Enterococcus spp.* and *E. coli* [6,18,26,38,41].

Non-typhoidal *Salmonella* (NTS) are among the most common bacteria isolated from foodborne infections of humans. Globally, there are approximately 94 million cases, including 155,000 deaths each year [1]. Animals are the most important reservoirs of NTS for humans [38,84–86]. Fecal shedding by carrier animals is an important source of antimicrobial resistant *Salmonella* contamination of meat and poultry products [38], and may also be responsible for fruit and vegetable contamination through fecal contamination of the environment [87]. *Salmonella* resistance to any medically important antimicrobial is of concern, but particularly to those critically important to human health, such as cephalosporins and fluoroquinolones [38,41,56]. Therapy in some groups (e.g., children and pregnant women) can be very restricted and beta-lactams such as third generation cephalosporins often may be the only therapy available to treat serious infections.

From the One Health antimicrobial resistance perspective, the third generation cephalosporins are good examples of antimicrobials that are considered critically important for both human and animal health. The main concern regarding selection and spread of resistance from animals to humans is their use as mass medications in large numbers of animals, either for therapy or prophylaxis. There are parallels with fluoroquinolones, another class of critically important antimicrobials, to which resistance among *Campylobacter jejuni* emerged following mass medication of poultry flocks [88–90]. In Australia where fluoroquinolones were never approved in food animals, fluoroquinolone resistant strains in food animals remain very rare [91].

Fluoroquinolone use in food animals is also linked to quinolone resistance in *Salmonella* [41,92–94]. Surveillance data compiled by WHO indicate that rates of fluoroquinolone resistance in non-typhoidal *Salmonella* vary widely by geographical region. For example, rates are relatively low in Europe (2–3%), higher in the Eastern Mediterranean region (up to 40–50%) and wide ranging in the Americas (0–96%) (1). Many *Salmonella* are also resistant to antimicrobials that have long been used as growth promoters in many countries (e.g., Canada, USA) including tetracyclines, penicillins and sulfonamides [41,84]. Antimicrobial resistance in some of the more virulent *Salmonella* serovars (e.g., Heidelberg, Newport, Typhimurium) has been associated with more severe infections in humans [38,83,86,95]. Resistance to other critically important antimicrobials continues to emerge in *Salmonella*, for example, a carbapenem resistant strain of *Salmonella* was identified on a pig farm that routinely administered prophylactic cephalosporin (ceftiofur) to piglets [96].

Escherichia coli are important pathogens of both humans and animals. In humans, *E. coli* are a common cause of serious bacterial infections, including enteritis, urinary tract infection and bloodstream infections [97–99]. Currently in England the rate for blood stream infections is about 64 cases per 100,000 per year and rising. A large and increasing proportion involves antimicrobial resistance, including fluoroquinolone resistance [100]. These higher rates are also being seen in countries with good surveillance systems in place, for example Denmark [60].

Many *E. coli* appear to behave as commensals of the gut of animals and humans, but may be opportunistic pathogens as well as donors of resistance genetic elements for pathogenic *E. coli* or other species of bacteria [101,102]. Although antimicrobial resistance is a rapidly increasing problem in *E. coli* infections of both animals and humans, the problem is better documented for isolates from human infections, where resistance is extensive, particularly in developing countries [1,103]. Humans are regularly exposed to antimicrobial resistant *E. coli* through foods and inadequately treated drinking water [104,105].

Travelers from developed countries are at risk of acquiring multi-resistance *E. coli* from other people or contaminated food and/or water [97,105,106]. There are now serious problems with extended spectrum beta lactamase (ESBL) *E. coli* in both developing and developed countries and foods from animals, in particular poultry, have been implicated as sources for humans [99,107,108], although the magnitude of the contribution from food animals is uncertain [102–104].

Given the critical importance of third and fourth generation cephalosporins and fluoroquinolones to human medicine and the clear evidence that treatment of entire groups of animals selects for resistance in important pathogens that spread from animals to humans [56,90], these drugs should be used rarely, if at all in animals, and only when supporting laboratory data demonstrate that no suitable alternatives of lesser human health importance are available. Their use as mass medications should be restricted.

Serious staphylococcal infections in people are common, including with Methicillin-resistant *Staphylococcus aureus* (MRSA) in both community and hospital settings, causing skin, wound, bloodstream and other types of infection [1,109–111]. *Staphylococcus aureus* and other staphylococci are also recognized pathogens of animals, for example they are responsible for cases of mastitis in cattle, and skin infections in pigs and companion animals [112,113]. MRSA were until recently relatively rare in animals but strains pathogenic to humans have emerged in several animal species [113–116]. Transmission to humans is thought currently to be mainly through contact with carrier animals [116]. The predominant strain isolated from animals is sequence type (ST) 398, and while pathogenic to humans, it is not considered a major epidemic strain [112,113]. Antimicrobial use in livestock, as well as lapses in biosecurity within and between farms, and international trade in animals, food or other products, are factors contributing to the spread of this pathogen in animals [113,117].

5. One Health Considerations from the Environment

One Health includes consideration of the environment as well as human and animal health [23,111]. The ecological nature of antimicrobial resistance is a reflection and consequence of the interconnectedness and diversity of life on the planet [22]. Many pathogenic bacteria, the antimicrobials that we use to treat them, and genes that confer resistance, have environmental origins (e.g., soil) [8,14,20]. Some important resistance genes, such as beta lactamases, are millions of years old [14,15]. Soil and other environmental matrices are rich sources of highly diverse populations of bacteria and their genes [14,118]. Antimicrobial resistance to a wide variety of drugs has been demonstrated in environmental bacteria isolated from the pre-antibiotic era, as well as from various sites (e.g., caves) free of other sources of exposure to modern antimicrobials [8,15,111,119]. Despite having ancient origins, there is abundant evidence that human activity has an impact on the resistome, which is the totality of resistance genes in the wider environment [13,14,118,119]. Hundreds of thousands of tons of antimicrobials are produced annually and find their way into the environment [18,27]. Waste from treatment plants and pharmaceutical industry, particularly if inadequately treated, can release high concentrations of antimicrobials into surface water [18,19,120,121]. Residues of antimicrobials are constituents of human sewage, livestock manure, and aquaculture, along with fecal bacteria and resistance genes [118,122–125]. Sewage treatment and composting of manure reduce concentrations of some but not all antimicrobials and microorganisms, which are introduced to soil upon land application of human and animal bio-solids [126].

Various environmental pathways are important routes of human exposure to resistant bacteria and their genes from animal and plant reservoirs [18,96,127] and provide opportunities for better regulations to control antimicrobial resistance. In developed countries with good quality sewage and drinking water treatment, and where most people have little to no direct contact with food-producing animals, transmission of bacteria and resistance genes from agricultural sources is largely foodborne, either from direct contamination of meat and poultry during slaughter and processing, or indirectly from fruit and vegetables contaminated by manure or irrigation water [38,87,90].

In countries with poor sewage and water treatment, drinking water is likely to be very important in transmission of resistant bacteria and/or genes from animals [11,97,111,120]). Poor sanitation also facilitates indirect person–person waterborne transmission of enteric bacteria among residents as well as international travelers who then return home colonized with resistant bacteria acquired locally [103,128]. Through these and other means, including globalized trade in animals and food, and long-distance migratory patterns of wildlife, antimicrobial resistant bacteria are globally disseminated.

General measures to address antimicrobial resistance in the wider environment include improved controls on pollution from industrial, residential and agricultural sources. Improved research as well as environmental monitoring and risk assessment is required to better understand the role of the environment in selection and spread of antimicrobial resistance, and to identify more specific measures to address resistance in this sector [12,14,18,100,103,129].

6. One Health Strategies to Address Antimicrobial Resistance

WHO and other international agencies (e.g., Food and Agriculture Organization (FAO), World Organization for Animal Health (OIE)), along with many individual countries, have developed comprehensive action plans to address the antimicrobial resistance crisis [5,130–136]. The WHO Global Action Plan seeks to address five major objectives that comprise the subtitles of the following sections. The WHO Plan embraces a One Health approach to address antimicrobial resistance, and it calls on member countries to do the same when developing their own action plans (6). There are five main pillars to the WHO Global Plan:

1. Improve Awareness and Understanding of Antimicrobial Resistance through Effective Communication, Education and Training
2. Strengthen the Knowledge and Evidence Base through Surveillance and Research
3. Reduce the Incidence of Infection through Effective Sanitation, Hygiene and Infection Prevention Measures
4. Optimize the Use of Antimicrobial Medicines in Human and Animal Health
5. Develop the Economic Case tor Sustainable Investment that Takes Account of the Needs of All Countries, and Increase Investment in New Medicines, Diagnostic Tools, Vaccines and Other Interventions

The One Health approach laid out in the WHO Global Action Plan is appropriate and consistent with statements made in action plans from other international and national organizations. There is however, a long way to go before a fully integrated One Health approach to antimicrobial resistance is implemented at country and global levels. Among the numerous barriers to overcome include the competing interests among multiple sectors (involving animals, humans, and environment) and organizations, agreement on priorities for action, and gaps in antimicrobial resistance surveillance, antimicrobial use policy, and infection control in many parts of the world.

7. Conclusions

History has shown that it is not feasible to neatly separate antimicrobial classes into those exclusively for use in human or non-human sectors, with the exception of new antimicrobial classes. These should probably be reserved for use in humans as long as there are few or no alternatives available. The majority of classes, however, will be available for use in both sectors and the challenge for One Health is to ensure that use of these drugs is optimal overall. This is likely to be achieved when antimicrobials used in both sectors are used for therapy, only rarely for prophylaxis and never for growth promotion, and when we better control the types and amounts of antimicrobials plus the numbers of resistant bacteria we allow to be placed into the environment. What is vitally important is that we do more to stop the spread of resistant bacteria—not only from person to person but between and within the human and agriculture sectors and the environment, giving particular emphasis to controls of contaminated water.

Funding: This research received no external funding.

Conflicts of Interest: The authors declare no conflict of interest.

References

1. World Health Organization (WHO). *Antimicrobial Resistance: Global Report on Surveillance*; WHO: Geneva, Switzerland, 2014.
2. Centers for Disease Control (CDC). *Antibiotic Resistance Threats in the United States*; CDC: Atlanta, GA, USA, 2013.
3. O'Neill, J. Tackling Drug-Resistant Infections Globally: Final Report and Recommendations the Review On Antimicrobial Resistance. 2016. Available online: https://amr-review.org/sites/default/files/160525_Finalpaper_withcover.pdf (accessed on 15 January 2019).
4. Laxminarayan, R.; Duse, A.; Wattal, C.; Zaidi, A.K.M.; Wertheim, H.F.L.; Sumpradit, N.; Vlieghe, E.; Hara, G.L.; Gould, I.M.; Goossens, H.; et al. Antibiotic Resistance—The Need for Global Solutions. *Lancet Infect. Dis.* **2013**, *13*, 1057–1098. [CrossRef]
5. World Health Organization (WHO). *Global Action Plan on Antimicrobial Resistance*; WHO: Geneva, Switzerland, 2015. Available online: http://www.wpro.who.int/entity/drug_resistance/resources/global_action_plan_eng.pdf (accessed on 15 January 2019).
6. Aarestrup, F.M.; Wegener, H.C.; Collignon, P. Resistance in Bacteria of The Food Chain: Epidemiology and Control Strategies. *Expert Rev. Anti-Infect. Ther.* **2008**, *6*, 733–750. [CrossRef]
7. Collignon, P.; Beggs, J.J.; Walsh, T.R.; Gandra, S.; Laxminarayan, R. Anthropological and Socioeconomic Factors Contributing to Global Antimicrobial Resistance: A Univariate and Multivariable Analysis. *Lancet Planet Heal.* **2018**, *2*, e398–e405. [CrossRef]
8. Holmes, A.H.; Moore, L.S.P.; Sundsfjord, A.; Steinbakk, M.; Regmi, S.; Karkey, A.; Guerin, P.J.; Piddock, L.J. Understanding the Mechanisms and Drivers of Antimicrobial Resistance. *Lancet* **2016**, *387*, 176–187. [CrossRef]
9. Burow, E.; Käsbohrer, A. Risk Factors for Antimicrobial Resistance in *Escherichia coli* in Pigs Receiving Oral Antimicrobial Treatment: A Systematic Review. *Microb. Drug Resist.* **2017**, *23*, 194–205. [CrossRef] [PubMed]
10. Marti, E.; Variatza, E.; Balcazar, J.L. The Role of Aquatic Ecosystems as Reservoirs of Antibiotic Resistance. *Trends Microbiol.* **2014**, *22*, 36–41. [CrossRef]
11. Bürgmann, H.; Frigon, D.; Gaze, W.H.; Manaia, C.M.; Pruden, A.; Singer, A.C.; Smets, B.F.; Zhang, T. Water and Sanitation: An Essential Battlefront in the War on Antimicrobial Resistance. *FEMS Microbiol. Ecol.* **2018**, *94*, fiy101. [CrossRef]
12. Huijbers, P.M.C.; Blaak, H.; de Jong, M.C.M.; Graat, E.A.M.; Vandenbroucke-Grauls, C.M.J.E.; de Roda Husman, A.M. Role of the Environment in the Transmission of Antimicrobial Resistance to Humans: A Review. *Environ. Sci. Technol.* **2015**, *49*, 11993–12004. [CrossRef]
13. Anonymous. Initiatives for Addressing Antimicrobial Resistance in the Environment: Current Situation and Challenges. 2018. Available online: https://wellcome.ac.uk/sites/default/files/antimicrobial-resistance-environment-report.pdf (accessed on 15 January 2019).
14. Gaze, W.H.; Krone, S.M.; Larsson, D.G.J.; Li, X.-Z.; Robinson, J.A.; Simonet, P.; Smalla, K.; Timinouni, M.; Topp, E.; Wellington, E.M.; et al. Influence of Humans on Evolution and Mobilization of Environmental Antibiotic Resistome. *Emerg. Infect. Dis.* **2013**, *19*, e120871. [CrossRef]
15. Perry, J.A.; Wright, G.D. Forces Shaping the Antibiotic Resistome. *BioEssays* **2014**, *36*, 1179–1184. [CrossRef]
16. Woolhouse, M.E.J.; Ward, M.J. Sources of Antimicrobial Resistance. *Science* **2013**, *341*, 1460–1461. [CrossRef]
17. Heuer, O.E.; Kruse, H.; Grave, K.; Collignon, P.; Karunasagar, I.; Angulo, F.J. Human Health Consequences of Use of Antimicrobial Agents in Aquaculture. *Clin. Infect. Dis.* **2009**, *49*, 1248–1253. [CrossRef]
18. O'Neill, J. Antimicrobials in Agriculture and the Environment: Reducing Unnecessary Use and Waste. The Review on Antimicrobial Resistance. 2015. Available online: https://amr-review.org/sites/default/files/Antimicrobialsinagricultureandtheenvironment---Reducingunnecessaryuseandwaste.pdf (accessed on 15 January 2019).
19. So, A.D.; Shah, T.A.; Roach, S.; Ling Chee, Y.; Nachman, K.E. An Integrated Systems Approach is Needed to Ensure the Sustainability of Antibiotic Effectiveness for Both Humans and Animals. *J. Law Med. Ethics* **2015**, *43*, 38–45. [CrossRef] [PubMed]

20. Collignon, P. The Importance of a One Health Approach to Preventing the Development and Spread of Antibiotic Resistance. In *One Health: The Human-Animal-Environment Interfaces in Emerging Infectious Diseases: Food Safety and Security, and International and National Plans for Implementation of One Health Activities*; Mackenzie, J.S., Jeggo, M., Daszak, P., Richt, J.A., Eds.; Springer: Berlin/Heidelberg, Germany, 2013; pp. 19–36.

21. Torren-Edo, J.; Grave, K.; Mackay, D. "One Health": The Regulation and Consumption of Antimicrobials for Animal Use in the EU. *IHAJ* **2015**, *2*, 14–16.

22. Robinson, T.P.; Bu, D.P.; Carrique-Mas, J.; Fèvre, E.M.; Gilbert, M.; Grace, D.; Hay, S.I.; Jiwakanon, J.; Kakkar, M.; Kariuki, S.; et al. Antibiotic Resistance is the Quintessential One Health Issue. *Trans. R. Soc. Trop. Med. Hyg.* **2016**, *110*, 377–380. [CrossRef] [PubMed]

23. Zinsstag, J.; Meisser, A.; Schelling, E.; Bonfoh, B.; Tanner, M. From 'Two Medicines' to 'One Health' and Beyond. *Onderstepoort J. Vet. Res.* **2012**, *79*, a492. [CrossRef]

24. World Health Organization. One Health. 2017. Available online: https://www.who.int/features/qa/one-health/en/ (accessed on 15 January 2019).

25. One Health Commission. What is One Health? 2018. Available online: https://www.onehealthcommission.org/en/why_one_health/what_is_one_health/ (accessed on 15 January 2019).

26. McEwen, S.A.; Fedorka-Cray, P.J. Antimicrobial Use and Resistance in Animals. *Clin. Infect. Dis.* **2002**, *34*, S93–S106. [CrossRef]

27. Van Boeckel, T.P.; Brower, C.; Gilbert, M.; Grenfell, B.T.; Levin, S.A.; Robinson, T.P.; Teillant, A.; Laxminarayan, R. Global Trends in Antimicrobial Use in Food Animals. *Proc. Natl. Acad. Sci. USA* **2015**, *112*, 5649–5654. [CrossRef]

28. European Medicines Agency (EMA). *Sales of Veterinary Antimicrobial Agents in 29 European Countries in 2014*; EMA: London, UK, 2016.

29. ECDC (European Centre for Disease Prevention and Control); EFSA (European Food Safety Authority); EMA (European Medicines Agency). ECDC/EFSA/EMA First Joint Report on The Integrated Analysis of The Consumption of Antimicrobial Agents and Occurrence of Antimicrobial Resistance in Bacteria from Humans and Food-Producing Animals. *EFSA J.* **2015**, *13*, 4006. [CrossRef]

30. Food and Agriculture Organization (FAO). Drivers, Dynamics and Epidemiology of Antimicrobial Resistance in Animal Oroduction. 2016. Available online: http://www.fao.org/3/a-i6209e.pdf (accessed on 15 January 2019).

31. Vidaver, A.K. Uses of Antimicrobials in Plant Agriculture. *Clin. Infect. Dis.* **2002**, *34*, S107–S110. [CrossRef]

32. Sundin, G.W.; Wang, N. Antibiotic Resistance in Plant-Pathogenic Bacteria. *Annu. Rev. Phytopathol.* **2018**, *56*, 161–180. [CrossRef] [PubMed]

33. Collignon, P. Use of Critically Important Antimicrobials in Food Production. In *Kucers' The Use of Antibiotics: A Clinical Review of Antibacterial, Antifungal, Antiparasitic and Antiviral Drugs*, 7th ed.; Grayson, L., Ed.; American Society for Microbiology and CRC Press: Boca Raton, FL, USA, 2018; pp. 9–18.

34. Sykes, J.E. Antimicrobial Drug Use in Dogs and Cats. In *Antimicrobial Therapy in Veterinary Medicine*, 5th ed.; Giguère, S., Prescott, J.F., Dowling, P.M., Eds.; John Wiley & Sons, Inc.: Hoboken, NJ, USA, 2013; pp. 473–494.

35. Giguère, S.; Abrams-Ogg, A.C.G.; Kruth, S.A. Prophylactic Use of Antimicrobial Agents, and Antimicrobial Chemotherapy for the Neutropenic Patient. In *Antimicrobial Therapy in Veterinary Medicine*, 5th ed.; Giguère, S., Prescott, J.F., Dowling, P.M., Eds.; John Wiley & Sons, Inc.: Hoboken, NJ, USA, 2013; pp. 357–378.

36. National Research Council. *The Use of Drugs in Food Animals: Benefits and Risks*; The National Academies Press: Washington, DC, USA, 1999.

37. Murphy, D.; Ricci, A.; Auce, Z.; Beechinor, J.G.; Bergendahl, H.; Breathnach, R.; Bures, J.; Pedro, J.; da Silva, D.; Hederová, J.; et al. EMA and EFSA Joint Scientific Opinion on Measures to Reduce the Need to Use Antimicrobial Agents in Animal Husbandry in the European Union, and the Resulting Impacts on Food Safety (RONAFA). *EFSA J.* **2017**, *15*, 4666.

38. Food and Agriculture Organization (FAO); World Organisation for Animal Health (OIE); World Health Organization (WHO) (FAO/OIE/WHO). *Joint FAO/OIE/WHO Expert Workshop on Non-Human Antimicrobial Usage and Antimicrobial Resistance: Scientific Assessment*; WHO: Geneva, Switzerland, 2003.

39. Food and Agriculture Organization (FAO); World Health Organization (WHO). *FAO/WHO Expert Meeting on Foodborne Antimicrobial Resistance: Role of Environment, Crops and Biocides. Summary Report*; FAO: Rome, Italy, 2018.

40. Zuraw, L. Perdue Announces Dramatic Reduction in Antibiotic Use in its Chickens. Food Safety News. 2014. Available online: http://www.foodsafetynews.com/2014/09/perdue-dramatically-reduces-antibiotic-use-in-chickens/#.WjLZulQ-dTZ (accessed on 15 January 2019).

41. World Health Organization (WHO). *Impacts of Antimicrobial Growth Promoter Termination in Denmark. The WHO International Review Panel's Evaluation of the Termination of the Use of Antimicrobial Growth Promoters in Denmark*; WHO: Foulum, Denmark, 2003.

42. World Health Organization (WHO). *The Medical Impact of the Use of Antimicrobials in Food Animals*; WHO: Berlin, Germany, 1997.

43. European Union (EU). Guidelines for the Prudent Use of Antimicrobials in Veterinary Medicine (2015/C 299/04). *Off. J. Eur. Union* **2015**, *C299*, C299:7–C299:26.

44. Food and Drug Administration (FDA). *Guidance for Industry #213. New Animal Drugs and New Animal Drug Combination Products Administered in or on Medicated Feed or Drinking Water of Food-Producing Animals: Recommendations for Drug Sponsors for Voluntarily Aligning Product Use Conditions with GFI #209*; FDA: Rockville, MD, USA, 2013.

45. Mehrotra, M.; Li, X.-Z.; Ireland, M.J. Enhancing Antimicrobial Stewardship by Strengthening the Veterinary Drug Regulatory Framework. *Can. Commun. Dis. Rep.* **2017**, *43*, 220–223. [CrossRef]

46. World Organisation for Animal Health (OIE). *OIE Annual Report on Antimicrobial Agents Intended for Use in Animals. Second Report*; OIE: Paris, France, 2018. Available online: http://www.oie.int/fileadmin/Home/eng/Our_scientific_expertise/docs/pdf/AMR/Annual_Report_AMR_2.pdf (accessed on 15 January 2019).

47. WHO Advisory Group on Integrated Surveillance of Antimicrobial Resistance (AGISAR). *Critically Important Antimicrobials for Human Medicine*; 4th revision 2013; World Health Organization: Geneva, Switzerland, 2016.

48. European Medicines Agency (EMA). *Revised Reflection Paper on the Use of 3rd and 4th Generation Cephalosporins in Food Producing Animals in the European Union: Development of Resistance and Impact on Human and Animal Health*; EMA: London, UK, 2009.

49. Prescott, J.F. Beta-lactam Antibiotics. In *Antimicrobial Therapy in Veterinary Medicine*, 5th ed.; Giguère, S., Prescott, J.F., Dowling, P.M., Eds.; John Wiley & Sons, Inc.: Hoboken, NJ, USA, 2013; pp. 153–173.

50. Food and Drug Administration (FDA). *2017 Summary Report on Antimicrobials Sold or Distributed for Use in Food-Producing Animals*; FDA: Washington, DC, USA, 2018.

51. Food and Drug Administration (FDA). *Drug Use Review. Food and Drug Administration, Department of Health and Human Services*; FDA: Washington, DC, USA, 2012. Available online: http://www.fda.gov/downloads/Drugs/DrugSafety/InformationbyDrugClass/UCM319435.pdf (accessed on 15 January 2019).

52. de Kraker, M.E.A.; Wolkewitz, M.; Davey, P.G.; Koller, W.; Berger, J.; Nagler, J.; Icket, C.; Kalenic, S.; Horvatic, J.; Seifert, H.; et al. Burden of Antimicrobial Resistance in European Hospitals: Excess Mortality and Length of Hospital Stay Associated with Bloodstream Infections due to *Escherichia coli* Resistant to Third-Generation Cephalosporins. *J. Antimicrob. Chemother.* **2011**, *66*, 398–407. [CrossRef]

53. Park, S.H. Third-Generation Cephalosporin Resistance in Gram-Negative Bacteria in the Community: A Growing Public Health Concern. *Korean J. Intern. Med.* **2014**, *29*, 27–30. [CrossRef] [PubMed]

54. Kanwar, N.; Scott, H.M.; Norby, B.; Loneragan, G.H.; Vinasco, J.; McGowan, M.; Cottell, J.L.; Chengappa, M.M.; Bai, J.; Boerlin, P. Effects of Ceftiofur and Chlortetracycline Treatment Strategies on Antimicrobial Susceptibility and on tet(A), tet(B), and blaCMY-2 Resistance Genes among *E. coli* Isolated from the Feces of Feedlot Cattle. *PLoS ONE* **2013**, *8*, e80575. [CrossRef]

55. Canadian Integrated Program for Antimicrobial Resistance (CIPARS). *Salmonella* Heidelberg—Ceftiofur-Related Resistance in Human and Retail Chicken Isolates. 2009. Available online: http://www.phac-aspc.gc.ca/cipars-picra/heidelberg/pdf/heidelberg_e.pdf (accessed on 15 January 2019).

56. Dutil, L.; Irwin, R.; Finley, R.; Ng, L.K.; Avery, B.; Boerlin, P.; Bourgault, A.M.; Cole, L.; Daignault, D.; Desruisseau, A.; et al. Ceftiofur Resistance in *Salmonella enterica* Serovar Heidelberg From Chicken Meat and Humans, Canada. *Emerg. Infect. Dis.* **2010**, *16*, 48–54. [CrossRef] [PubMed]

57. Smith, K.E.; Medus, C.; Meyer, S.D.; Boxrud, D.J.; Leano, F.; Hedberg, C.W.; Elfering, K.; Braymen, C.; Bender, J.B.; Danila, R.N. Outbreaks of Salmonellosis in Minnesota (1998 through 2006) Associated with Frozen, Microwaveable, Breaded, Stuffed Chicken Products. Vol. 71. *J. Food Prot.* **2008**, *71*, 2153–2160. [CrossRef] [PubMed]

58. Chicken Farmers of Canada. Antibiotics. 2018. Available online: https://www.chickenfarmers.ca/antibiotics/ (accessed on 15 January 2019).

59. Hiki, M.; Kawanishi, M.; Abo, H.; Kojima, A.; Koike, R.; Hamamoto, S.; Asai, T. Decreased Resistance to Broad-Spectrum Cephalosporin in *Escherichia coli* from Healthy Broilers at Farms in Japan After Voluntary Withdrawal of Ceftiofur. *Foodborne Pathog. Dis.* **2015**, *12*, 639–643. [CrossRef]

60. DANMAP 2014. Use of Antimicrobial Agents and Occurrence of Antimicrobial Resistance in Bacteria from Food Animals, Food and Humans in Denmark. Statens Serum Institut, National Veterinary Institute, Technical University of Denmark, National Food Institute, Technical University of Denmark, 2015. Available online: https://www.danmap.org/downloads/reports.aspx (accessed on 15 January 2019).

61. Department of Health and Human Services, Food and Drug Administration. 2012, 21 CFR Part 530 [Docket No. FDA–2008–N–0326] New Animal Drugs; Cephalosporin Drugs; Extra Label Animal Drug Use; Order of Prohibition. *Fed. Regist.* **2012**, *77*, 735–745.

62. European Medicines Agency (EMA). Answers to the Request for Scientific Advice on the Impact on Public Health and Animal Health of the Use of Antibiotics in Animals. 2014. Available online: http://www.ema.europa.eu/docs/en_GB/document_library/Other/2014/07/WC500170253.pdf (accessed on 15 January 2019).

63. European Medicines Agency (EMA). Updated Advice on the Use of Colistin Products in Animals Within the European Union: Development of Resistance and Possible Impact on Human and Animal Health. In *Committee for Medicinal Products for Veterinary use (CVMP), Committee for Medicinal Products*; EMA: London, UK, 2016.

64. Falagas, M.E.; Kasiakou, S.K. Toxicity of Polymyxins: A Systematic Review of the Evidence from Old and Recent Studies. *Crit. Care* **2006**, *10*, R27. [CrossRef] [PubMed]

65. Falagas, M.E.; Kasiakou, S.K.; Saravolatz, L.D. Colistin: The Revival of Polymyxins for the Management of Multidrug-Resistant Gram-Negative Bacterial Infections. *Clin. Infect. Dis.* **2005**, *40*, 1333–1341. [CrossRef] [PubMed]

66. Linden, P.K.; Kusne, S.; Coley, K.; Fontes, P.; Kramer, D.J.; Paterson, D. Use of Parenteral Colistin for the Treatment of Serious Infection Due to Antimicrobial-Resistant *Pseudomonas aeruginosa*. *Clin. Infect. Dis.* **2003**, *37*, e154–e160. [CrossRef]

67. Fernandes, M.R.; Moura, Q.; Sartori, L.; Silva, K.C.; Cunha, M.P.V.; Esposito, F.; Lopes, R.; Otutumi, L.K.; Gonçalves, D.D.; Dropa, M.; et al. Silent Dissemination of Colistin-Resistant *Escherichia coli* in South America Could Contribute to the Global Spread of the mcr-1 Gene. *Eurosurveillance* **2016**, *21*. [CrossRef]

68. Liu, Y.-Y.; Wang, Y.; Walsh, T.R.; Yi, L.-X.; Zhang, R.; Spencer, J.; Doi, Y.; Tian, G.; Dong, B.; Huang, X.; et al. Emergence of Plasmid-Mediated Colistin Rresistance Mechanism MCR-1 in Animals and Human Beings in China: A Microbiological and Molecular Biological Study. *Lancet Infect. Dis.* **2016**, *16*, 161–168. [CrossRef]

69. European Centers for Disease Control and Prevention (ECDC). *Summary of the Latest Data on Antibiotic Consumption in the European Union. Antibiotic Consumption in Europe*; ECDC: Stockholm, Sweden, 2015.

70. Landman, D.; Georgescu, C.; Martin, D.A.; Quale, J. Polymyxins Revisited. *Clin. Microbiol. Rev.* **2008**, *21*, 449–465. [CrossRef]

71. European Food Safety Authority (EFSA), European Centre for Disease Prevention and Control (ECDC). The European Union Summary Report on Antimicrobial Resistance in Zoonotic and Indicator Bacteria from Humans, Animals and Food in 2016. *EFSA J.* **2018**, *16*, e05182.

72. Catry, B.; Cavaleri, M.; Baptiste, K.; Grave, K.; Grein, K.; Holm, A.; Jukes, H.; Liebana, E.; Navas, A.L.; Mackay, D.; et al. Use of Colistin-Containing Products Within the European Union and European Economic Area (EU/EEA): Development of Resistance in Animals and Possible Impact on Human and Animal Health. *Int. J. Antimicrob Agents* **2015**, *46*, 297–306. [CrossRef]

73. Prim, N.; Rivera, A.; Rodríguez-Navarro, J.; Español, M.; Turbau, M.; Coll, P.; Mirelis, B. Detection of mcr-1 Colistin Resistance Gene in Polyclonal *Escherichia coli* Isolates in Barcelona, Spain, 2012 to 2015. *Eurosurveillance* **2016**, *21*. [CrossRef]

74. Irrgang, A.; Roschanski, N.; Tenhagen, B.-A.; Grobbel, M.; Skladnikiewicz-Ziemer, T.; Thomas, K.; Roesler, U.; Käsbohrer, A. Prevalence of mcr-1 in E. coli from Livestock and Food in Germany, 2010–2015. *PLoS ONE* **2016**, *11*, e0159863. [CrossRef]

75. Hasman, H.; Hammerum, A.M.; Hansen, F.; Hendriksen, R.S.; Olesen, B.; Agersø, Y.; Zankari, E.; Leekitcharoenphon, P.; Stegger, M.; Kaas, R.S.; et al. Detection of mcr-1 Encoding Plasmid-Mediated Colistin-Resistant *Escherichia coli* Isolates from Human Bloodstream Infection and Imported Chicken Meat, Denmark 2015. *Eurosurveillance* **2015**, *20*. [CrossRef] [PubMed]

76. Wang, R.; van Dorp, L.; Shaw, L.P.; Bradley, P.; Wang, Q.; Wang, X.; Jin, L.; Zhang, Q.; Liu, Y.; Rieux, A.; et al. The Global Distribution and Spread of the Mobilized Colistin Resistance Gene mcr-1. *Nat. Commun.* **2018**, *9*, 1179. [CrossRef]

77. von Wintersdorff, C.J.H.; Wolffs, P.F.G.; van Niekerk, J.M.; Beuken, E.; van Alphen, L.B.; Stobberingh, E.E.; Oude Lashof, A.M.L.; Hoebe, C.J.P.A.; Savelkoul, P.H.M.; Penders, J. Detection of the Plasmid-Mediated Colistin-Resistance Gene mcr-1 in Faecal Metagenomes of Dutch Travellers. *J. Antimicrob Chemother.* **2016**, *71*, 3416–3419. [CrossRef]

78. Shen, Z.; Wang, Y.; Shen, Y.; Shen, J.; Wu, C. Early Emergence of mcr-1 in *Escherichia coli* from Food-Producing Animals. *Lancet Infect. Dis.* **2016**, *16*, 293. [CrossRef]

79. Zurfuh, K.; Poirel, L.; Nordmann, P.; Nüesch-Inderbinen, M.; Hächler, H.; Stephan, R. Occurrence of the Plasmid-Borne mcr-1 Colistin Resistance Gene in Extended-Spectrum-β-Lactamase-Producing Enterobacteriaceae in River Water and Imported Vegetable Samples in Switzerland. *Antimicrob. Agents Chemother.* **2016**, *60*, 2594–2595. [CrossRef] [PubMed]

80. Xavier, B.B.; Lammens, C.; Ruhal, R.; Kumar-Singh, S.; Butaye, P.; Goossens, H.; Malhotra-Kumar, S. Identification of a Novel Plasmid-Mediated Colistin-Resistance Gene, mcr-2, in *Escherichia coli*, Belgium, June 2016. *Eurosurveillance* **2016**, *21*. [CrossRef]

81. Levine, D.P. Vancomycin: A History. *Clin. Infect. Dis.* **2006**, *42*, S5–S12. [CrossRef]

82. Bager, F.; Madsen, M.; Christensen, J.; Aarestrup, F.M. Avoparcin Used as a Growth Promoter is Associated with the Occurrence of Vancomycin-Resistant *Enterococcus faecium* on Danish Poultry and Pig Farms. *Prev. Vet. Med.* **1997**, *31*, 95–112. [CrossRef]

83. Barza, M. Potential Mechanisms of Increased Disease in Humans from Antimicrobial Resistance in Food Animals. *Clin. Infect. Dis.* **2002**, *34*, S123–S125. [CrossRef]

84. Anderson, E.S. Drug Resistance in *Salmonella typhimurium* and its Implications. *Br. Med. J.* **1968**, *3*, 333–339. [CrossRef] [PubMed]

85. Swann, M.M. *The Use of Antibiotics in Animal Husbandry and Veterinary Medicine*; HMSO: London, UK, 1969.

86. Institute of Medicine. *Human Health Risks with the Subtherapeutic Use of Penicillin or Tetracyclines in Animal Feed*; The National Academies Press: Washington, DC, USA, 1989.

87. Hanning, I.B.; Nutt, J.D.; Ricke, S.C. Salmonellosis Outbreaks in the United States Due to Fresh Produce: Sources and Potential Intervention Measures. *Foodborne Pathog. Dis.* **2009**, *6*, 635–648. [CrossRef] [PubMed]

88. Endtz, H.; Ruijs, G.; van Klingeren, B.; Jansen, W.H.; Reijden, T.; Mouton, R.P. Quinolone Resistance in *Campylobacter* Isolated from Man and Poultry Following the Introduction of Fluoroquinolones in Veterinary Medicine. *J. Antimicrob Chemother.* **1991**, *27*, 199–208. [CrossRef] [PubMed]

89. McDermott, P.F.; Bodeis, S.M.; English, L.L.; White, D.G.; WalkeR, R.D.; Zhao, S.; Simjee, S.; Wagne, D.D. Ciprofloxacin Resistance in *Campylobacter jejuni* Evolves Rapidly in Chickens Treated with Fluoroquinolones. *J. Infect. Dis.* **2002**, *185*, 837–840. [CrossRef]

90. Nelson, J.M.; Chiller, T.M.; Powers, J.H.; Angulo, F.J. Fluoroquinolone-Resistant *Campylobacter Species* and the Withdrawal of Fluoroquinolones from Use in Poultry: A Public Health Success Story. *Clin. Infect. Dis.* **2007**, *44*, 977–980. [CrossRef] [PubMed]

91. Cheng, A.C.; Turnidge, J.; Collignon, P.; Looke, D.; Barton, M.; Gottlieb, T. Control of Fluoroquinolone Resistance through Successful Regulation, Australia. *Emerg. Infect. Dis.* **2012**, *18*, 1453–1460. [CrossRef]

92. World Health Organization (WHO). *Use of Quinolones in Food Animals and Potential Impact on Human Health*; WHO: Geneva, Switzerland, 1998.

93. Chiu, C.H.; Wu, T.L.; Su, L.H.; Chu, C.; Chia, J.H.; Kuo, A.J.; Chien, M.S.; Lin, T.Y. The Emergence in Taiwan of Fluoroquinolone Resistance in *Salmonella enterica* Serotype Choleraesuis. *N. Engl. J. Med.* **2002**, *346*, 413–419. [CrossRef] [PubMed]

94. European Medicines Agency (EMA). *Reflection Paper on the Use of Fluoroquinolones in Food-Producing Animals in the European Union: Development of Resistance and Impact on Human and Animal Health*; EMEA/CVMP/SAGAM/184651/2005; EMA: London, UK, 2006.

95. Helms, M.; Simonsen, J.; Mølbak, K. Quinolone Resistance Is Associated with Increased Risk of Invasive Illness or Death during Infection with *Salmonella* Serotype Typhimurium. *J. Infect. Dis.* **2004**, *190*, 1652–1654. [CrossRef] [PubMed]

96. Mollenkopf, D.F.; Stull, J.W.; Mathys, D.A.; Bowman, A.S.; Feicht, S.M.; Grooters, S.V.; Daniels, J.B.; Wittum, T.E. Carbapenemase-Producing Enterobacteriaceae Recovered from the Environment of a Swine Farrow-to-Finish Operation in the United States. *Antimicrob. Agents Chemother.* **2017**, *61*, e01298-16. [CrossRef] [PubMed]

97. Kennedy, K.; Collignon, P. Colonisation with *Escherichia coli* Resistant to "Critically Important" Antibiotics: A High Risk for International Travellers. *Eur. J. Clin. Microbiol. Infect. Dis.* **2010**, *29*, 1501–1506. [CrossRef]

98. Laupland, K.B.; Church, D.L. Population-Based Epidemiology and Microbiology of Community-Onset Bloodstream Infections. *Clin. Microbiol. Rev.* **2014**, *27*, 647–664. [CrossRef] [PubMed]

99. Lazarus, B.; Paterson, D.L.; Mollinger, J.L.; Rogers, B.A. Do Human Extraintestinal *Escherichia coli* Infections Resistant to Expanded-Spectrum Cephalosporins Originate From Food-Producing Animals? A Systematic Review. *Clin. Infect. Dis.* **2015**, *60*, 439–452. [CrossRef] [PubMed]

100. Bou-Antoun, S.; Davies, J.; Guy, R.; Johnson, A.P.; Sheridan, E.A.; Hope, R.J. Descriptive Epidemiology of *Escherichia coli* Bacteraemia in England, April 2012 to March 2014. *Eurosurveillance* **2016**, *21*. [CrossRef] [PubMed]

101. Hammerum, A.M.; Larsen, J.; Andersen, V.D.; Lester, C.H.; Skovgaard Skytte, T.S.; Hansen, F.; Olsen, S.S.; Mordhorst, H.; Skov, R.L.; Aarestrup, F.M.; et al. Characterization of Extended-Spectrum β-lactamase (ESBL)-Producing *Escherichia coli* Obtained from Danish Pigs, Pig farmers and Their Families from Farms with High or no Consumption of Third- or Fourth-Generation Cephalosporins. *J. Antimicrob Chemother.* **2014**, *69*, 2650–2657. [CrossRef] [PubMed]

102. Collignon, P. Antibiotic Resistance: Are we all Doomed? *Intern. Med. J.* **2015**, *45*, 1109–1115. [CrossRef]

103. Walsh, T.R.; Weeks, J.; Livermore, D.M.; Toleman, M.A. Dissemination of NDM-1 positive Bacteria in the New Delhi Environment and its Implications for Human Health: An Environmental Point Prevalence Study. *Lancet Infect. Dis.* **2011**, *11*, 355–362. [CrossRef]

104. Graham, D.W.; Collignon, P.; Davies, J.; Larsson, D.G.J.; Snape, J. Underappreciated Role of Regionally Poor Water Quality on Globally Increasing Antibiotic Resistance. *Environ. Sci. Technol.* **2014**, *48*, 11746–11747. [CrossRef]

105. Tängdén, T.; Cars, O.; Melhus, Å.; Löwdin, E. Foreign Travel Is a Major Risk Factor for Colonization with *Escherichia coli* Producing CTX-M-Type Extended-Spectrum β-Lactamases: A Prospective Study with Swedish Volunteers. *Antimicrob. Agents Chemother.* **2010**, *54*, 3564–3568. [CrossRef]

106. Vieira, A.R.; Collignon, P.; Aarestrup, F.M.; McEwen, S.A.; Hendriksen, R.S.; Hald, T.; Wegener, H.C. Association Between Antimicrobial Resistance in *Escherichia coli* Isolates from Food Animals and Blood Stream Isolates From Humans in Europe: An Ecological Study. *Foodborne Pathog. Dis.* **2011**, *8*, 1295–1301. [CrossRef]

107. De Been, M.; Lanza, V.F.; de Toro, M.; Scharringa, J.; Dohmen, W.; Du, Y.; Hu, J.; Lei, Y.; Li, N.; Tooming-Klunderud, A.; et al. Dissemination of Cephalosporin Resistance Genes between *Escherichia coli* Strains from Farm Animals and Humans by Specific Plasmid Lineages. *PLOS Genet.* **2014**, *10*, e1004776. [CrossRef] [PubMed]

108. Jakobsen, L.; Kurbasic, A.; Skjøt-Rasmussen, L.; Ejrnæs, K.; Porsbo, L.J.; Pedersen, K.; Jensen, L.B.; Emborg, H.-D.; Agersø, Y.; Olsen, K.E.P.; et al. *Escherichia coli* Isolates from Broiler Chicken Meat, Broiler Chickens, Pork, and Pigs Share Phylogroups and Antimicrobial Resistance with Community-Dwelling Humans and Patients with Urinary Tract Infection. *Foodborne Pathog. Dis.* **2009**, *7*, 537–547. [CrossRef] [PubMed]

109. ECDC (European Centre for Disease Prevention and Control); EFSA (European Food Safety Authority); EMA (European Medicines Agency). Joint Scientific Report of ECDC, EFSA and EMEA on Meticillin Resistant *Staphylococcus aureus* (MRSA) in Livestock, Companion Animals and Food. *EFSA J.* **2009**, *7*. [CrossRef]

110. European Centre for Disease Prevention and Control (ECDC). *Antimicrobial Resistance Surveillance in Europe 2014. Annual Report of the European Antimicrobial Resistance Surveillance Network (EARS-Net)*; ECDC: Stockholm, Sweden, 2015.

111. Finley, R.L.; Collignon, P.; Larsson, D.G.J.; McEwen, S.A.; Li, X.-Z.; Gaze, W.H.; Reid-Smith, R.; Timinouni, M.; Graham, D.W.; Topp, E. The Scourge of Antibiotic Resistance: The Important Role of the Environment. *Clin. Infect. Dis.* **2013**, *57*, 704–710. [CrossRef] [PubMed]

112. Price, L.B.; Stegger, M.; Hasman, H.; Aziz, M.; Larsen, J.; Andersen, P.S.; Pearson, T.; Waters, A.E.; Foster, J.T.; Schupp, J.; et al. *Staphylococcus aureus* CC398: Host Adaptation and Emergence of Methicillin Resistance in Livestock. *mBio* **2012**, e00305-11. [CrossRef] [PubMed]

113. Weese, J.S.; van Duijkeren, E. Methicillin-Resistant *Staphylococcus aureus* and *Staphylococcus pseudintermedius* in Veterinary Medicine. *Vet. Microbiol.* **2010**, *140*, 418–429. [CrossRef] [PubMed]

114. Boost, M.V.; O'Donoghue, M.M.; Siu, K.H.G. Characterisation of Methicillin-Resistant *Staphylococcus aureus* Isolates from Dogs and Their Owners. *Clin. Microbiol. Infect.* **2007**, *13*, 731–733. [CrossRef]

115. Lewis, H.C.; Mølbak, K.; Reese, C.; Aarestrup, F.M.; Selchau, M.; Sørum, M.; Skov, R.L. Pigs as Source of Methicillin-Resistant *Staphylococcus aureus* CC398 Infections in Humans, Denmark. *Emerg. Infect. Dis.* **2008**, *14*, 1383–1389. [CrossRef]

116. Voss, A.; Loeffen, F.; Bakker, J.; Klaassen, C.; Wulf, M. Methicillin-Resistant *Staphylococcus aureus* in Pig Farming. *Emerg. Infect. Dis. J.* **2005**, *11*, 1965. [CrossRef]

117. Dorado-Garcia, A.; Dohmen, W.; Bos, M.E.H.; Verstappen, K.M.; Houben, M.; Wagenaar, J.A.; Heederik, D.J. Dose-Response Relationship Between Antimicrobial Drugs and Livestock-Associated MRSA in Pig Farming. *Emerg. Infect. Dis.* **2015**, *21*, 950–959. [CrossRef]

118. Ruuskanen, M.; Muurinen, J.; Meierjohan, A.; Parnanen, K.; Tamminen, M.; Lyra, C.; Kronberg, L.; Virta, M. Fertilizing with Animal Manure Disseminates Antibiotic Resistance Genes to the Farm Environment. *J. Environ. Qual.* **2016**, *45*, 488–493. [CrossRef]

119. Wellington, E.M.H.; Boxall, A.B.; Cross, P.; Feil, E.J.; Gaze, W.H.; Hawkey, P.M.; Johnson-Rollings, A.S.; Jones, D.L.; Lee, N.M.; Otten, W.; et al. The Role of the Natural Environment in the Emergence of Antibiotic Resistance in Gram-Negative Bacteria. *Lancet Infect. Dis.* **2013**, *13*, 155–165. [CrossRef]

120. Aubertheau, E.; Stalder, T.; Mondamert, L.; Ploy, M.-C.; Dagot, C.; Labanowski, J. Impact of Wastewater Treatment Plant Discharge on the Contamination of River Biofilms by Pharmaceuticals and Antibiotic Resistance. *Sci. Total Environ.* **2017**, *579*, 1387–1398. [CrossRef]

121. Singer, A.C.; Shaw, H.; Rhodes, V.; Hart, A. Review of Antimicrobial Resistance in the Environment and Its Relevance to Environmental Regulators. *Front. Microbiol.* **2016**, *7*, 1728. [CrossRef] [PubMed]

122. Rizzo, L.; Manaia, C.; Merlin, C.; Schwartz, T.; Dagot, C.; Ploy, M.C.; Michael, I.; Fatta-Kassinos, D. Urban Wastewater Treatment Plants as Hotspots for Antibiotic Resistant Bacteria and Genes Spread into the Environment: A Review. *Sci. Total Environ.* **2013**, *447*, 345–360. [CrossRef]

123. Zhang, Q.-Q.; Ying, G.-G.; Pan, C.-G.; Liu, Y.-S.; Zhao, J.-L. Comprehensive Evaluation of Antibiotics Emission and Fate in the River Basins of China: Source Analysis, Multimedia Modeling, and Linkage to Bacterial Resistance. *Environ. Sci. Technol.* **2015**, *49*, 6772–6782. [CrossRef] [PubMed]

124. Cabello, F.C.; Godfrey, H.P.; Buschmann, A.H.; Dölz, H.J. Aquaculture as yet Another Environmental Gateway to the Development and Globalisation of Antimicrobial Resistance. *Lancet Infect. Dis.* **2016**, *16*, e127–e133. [CrossRef]

125. Wang, H.; Yang, J.; Yu, X.; Zhao, G.; Zhao, Q.; Wang, N.; Jiang, Y.; Jiang, F.; He, G.; Chen, Y.; et al. Exposure of Adults to Antibiotics in a Shanghai Suburban Area and Health Risk Assessment: A Biomonitoring-Based Study. *Environ. Sci. Technol.* **2018**, *52*, 13942–13950. [CrossRef]

126. Rahube, T.O.; Marti, R.; Scott, A.; Tien, Y.-C.; Murray, R.; Sabourin, L.; Duenk, P.; Lapen, D.R.; Topp, E. Persistence of antibiotic resistance and plasmid-associated genes in soil following application of sewage sludge and abundance on vegetables at harvest. *Can. J. Microbiol.* **2016**, *62*, 600–607. [CrossRef]

127. European Medicines Agency (EMA). Reflection Paper on Antimicrobial Resistance in the Environment: Considerations for Current and Future Risk Assessment of Veterinary Medicinal Products Draft. 2018. Available online: https://www.ema.europa.eu/documents/scientific-guideline/draft-reflection-paper-antimicrobial-resistance-environment-considerations-current-future-risk_en.pdf (accessed on 15 January 2019).

128. Collignon, P.; Kennedy, K.J. Long-Term Persistence of Multidrug-Resistant Enterobacteriaceae after Travel. *Clin. Infect. Dis.* **2015**, *61*, 1766–1767. [CrossRef] [PubMed]

129. Ashbolt, N.J.; Amézquita, A.; Backhaus, T.; Borriello, P.; Brandt, K.K.; Collignon, P.; Coors, A.; Finley, R.; Gaze, W.H.; Heberer, T.; et al. Human Health Risk Assessment (HHRA) for Environmental Development and Transfer of Antibiotic Resistance. *Environ. Health Perspect.* **2013**, *121*, 993–1001. [CrossRef] [PubMed]

130. World Organisation for Animal Health (OIE). *The OIE Strategy on Antimicrobial Resistance and the Prudent Use of Antimicrobials*; OIE: Paris, France, 2016.

131. Department of Health and Department for Environment Food & Rural Affairs. *UK Five-Year Antimicrobial Resistance Strategy 2013 to 2018*; Department of Health and Department for Environment Food & Rural Affairs: London, UK, 2013.

132. Public Health Agency of Canada. *Federal Action Plan on Antimicrobial Resistance and Use in Canada*; Public Health Agency of Canada: Ottawa, ON, Cananda, 2015.

133. Commonwealth of Australia. *Responding to the Threat of Antimicrobial Resistance. Australia's First National Antimicrobial Resistance Strategy 2015-2019*; Commonwealth of Australia: Canberra, Australia, 2016.

134. European Union (EU). *Communication from the Commission to the European Parliament and the Council. Action Plan against the Rising Threats from Antimicrobial Resistance*; EU: Brussels, Belgium, 2011.

135. The White House. *National Action Plan for Combating Antibiotic-Resistant Bacteria*; The White House: Washington, DC, USA, 2015.

136. Food and Agriculture Organization (FAO). *The FAO Action Plan on Antimicrobial Resistance 2016-2020*; FAO: Rome, Italy, 2016.

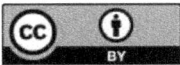

Tropical Medicine and Infectious Disease

MDPI

Commentary

Antimicrobial Resistance (AMR) in the Food Chain: Trade, One Health and Codex

Anna George [1,2]

[1] Centre on Global Health Security, Chatham House, London SW1Y 4LE, UK; anna.george.c@gmail.com or Anna.George@murdoch.edu.au
[2] Public Policy and International Affairs, Murdoch University, Murdoch, WA 6150, Australia

Received: 6 March 2019; Accepted: 22 March 2019; Published: 26 March 2019

Abstract: Strategies that take on a One Health approach to addressing antimicrobial resistance (AMR) focused on reducing human use of antimicrobials, but policy-makers now have to grapple with a different set of political, economic, and highly sensitive trade interests less amenable to government direction, to tackle AMR in the food chain. Understanding the importance and influence of the intergovernmental Codex negotiations underway on AMR in the Food Chain is very weak but essential for AMR public policy experts. National and global food producing industries are already under pressure as consumers learn about the use of antimicrobials in food production and more so when the full impact of AMR microorganisms in the food chain and on the human microbiome is better understood. Governments will be expected to respond. Trade-related negotiations on access and use made of antimicrobials is political: the relevance of AMR 'evidence' is already contested and not all food producers or users of antimicrobials in the food chain are prepared to, or capable of, moving at the same pace. In trade negotiations governments defend their interpretation of national interest. Given AMR in the global food chain threatens national interest, both AMR One Health and zoonotic disease experts should understand and participate in all trade-related AMR negotiations to protect One Health priorities. To help facilitate this an overview and analysis of Codex negotiations is provided.

Keywords: AMR; One Health; food chain; trade; Codex; WHO; World Trade Organization (WTO)

1. Background: Access to and Use of Antimicrobials

A global political consensus has been reached confirming antimicrobials underpin human health security so access and use of these miracle products has to be wound back across all sectors of the economy [1]. One key agenda slow to emerge is antimicrobial resistance in the food chain with consequences for food safety, food security and significant implications for trade policy.

The complex integrated strategies needed to reign-in the use of antimicrobials in the food, agricultural and associated industry sectors have the capacity to transform the somewhat benign and logical 'AMR (antimicrobial resistance) One Health Framework' into a quagmire of competing interests—as not all producers and users of antimicrobials are prepared to, and some not yet capable of, limiting their use of antimicrobials. But to preserve the AMR One Health global consensus much will depend on how these trade related issues are handled and will require significant leadership and clear recognition of the health security implications of failure.

The UK 2016 O'Neil AMR Report [2] mapped out possible consequences of not safeguarding these precious antimicrobials and analyzed the capacity of this AMR phenomena to economically disrupt and negatively impact on many industry sectors. On the human costs, more accurate research and analysis recording actual numbers of AMR related deaths and the exponential growth of health/productivity costs is emerging that will better reflect the consequences from AMR events [3,4]. This sensitive data is likely to reverberate politically.

Such politically sensitive data and revelations from research on AMR in the food chain will inevitably place 'food trade' firmly in the spotlight. Trade policy, at its best, can help induce higher safety standards, better quality food, and safer products. But the spread of AMR microorganisms could represent one of the biggest challenges to trade in safe food and may lead to trade disruption and financial loss.

Existing trade frameworks and obligations may be capable of addressing this issue but only if sensitized and adapted to prioritize safeguarding health security by providing the flexibility for governments to implement measures to safeguard their food-chain and help preserve antimicrobials, particularly those important for human medicine.

AMR is an economic and global trade issue, so criticism of government action or regulatory changes perceived as running counter to concepts of 'free trade' will need to be managed. But this is also an opportunity for those who have extolled the benefits of trade to step up and deliver on this crucial AMR agenda.

There are after all several precedents where similar large and economically painful transformations have been deemed necessary linked to 'access and use'—sometimes for the public or global good and often to facilitate trade in new technologies or facilitate new forms of production and accumulation. For example, intellectual property and copyright provisions extended through WTO Trade-Related Aspects of Intellectual Property (TRIPS) [5]; reducing chemical toxicity in domestic products—EU REACH Legislation (Registration, Evaluation, Authorization and Restrictions of Chemicals) [6], and promoting health objectives—Tobacco Plain Packaging Policy [7].

With such complex trade agendas, it was inevitably these transformations created economic disruption by altering access and or use provisions which redistributed costs, benefits, investments and profits. All involved high levels of political contestation as access provisions and/or regulations were redefined at the national level or through multilateral negotiations. Interestingly, lessons and tactics used to support or block these transformations are beginning to resonate in the AMR debates and some have been picked up by media [8].

Implementing effective AMR One Health strategies will require a similar level of political commitment and leadership to transform access and use provisions to preserve the efficacy of antimicrobials, particularly for human medicine.

2. Policy Coherence—Are Trade Policies Understood and Integrated into AMR One Health Strategies?

National AMR One Health Strategies already focus on altering both access provisions and use made of antimicrobials for human use. The other major area of antibiotic use—food production—is yet to be as systematically adapted to achieve national one health objectives. Unlike reducing human use which is negotiated and conducted entirely at the national level usually by government health authorities, but to influence the access and use of antimicrobials in food production (domestic and imported) is more complex. And involves many more interested parties. The 2006 EU ban on the use of antibiotics as growth promotors is an example of the complex legal, trade and political implications that can flow from such decisions.

A fundamental understanding how national trade policies harmonize/comply with international trade rules and obligations is essential. This includes understanding the technical and legal structures that enable and legitimize the use of antimicrobials in the food chain as well as the capacity to exclude them in specific circumstances from imported food.

This will require AMR public health experts to be active in setting AMR government priorities in these trade-related negotiations to ensure AMR policy coherence: The international standard setting body for food safety, Codex Alimentarius Commission (Codex); the World Trade Organization (WTO); and also Bilateral and Regional Free Trade Agreements.

The rational for engaging in such esoteric areas of trade policy is that any new interpretations, obligations, rules, procedures/guidelines evolving from, for example, Codex negotiations on 'AMR in the food chain' have the capacity to impact on the access to and use made of antimicrobials. But of equal importance, such multilateral decisions could also circumscribe the regulatory and legal options available to national governments in implementing their AMR strategies and their domestic export/import policies if national legislation/regulations are not introduced or adapted to reflect One Health priorities. One example to be aware of is introducing the capacity to develop 'national lists' of antimicrobials as discussed in Codex TFAMR Report REP 19/AMR.

An overview of negotiations currently underway in the Codex food standard setting body may help make transparent the complex political and legal obligations linked to international trade. Understanding the food/trade linkage is critical especially if national inter-agency policy cohesion has not fully integrated these trade-related elements. And introducing new regulations on AMR may be problematic if political commitment or bureaucratic capacity to regulate is weak.

For example, the technical and scientific complexity of the AMR/food subject matter and navigating the huge number of Codex standards and guidelines [9] is challenging so these negotiations are usually left to 'expert' bodies responsible for Codex, or, decisions driven by broader national trade objectives managed through foreign/trade policy negotiators.

Bureaucratically integrating the trade agenda into One Health Action Plans may be difficult but is essential. These trade-related linkages should be comprehensively understood for their effect and appropriately responded to in-line with national AMR One Health security priorities.

3. Codex Alimentarius Commission (Codex): Current Negotiations on AMR in the Food Chain and Understanding the Political Context

AMR in the food chain was earlier addressed through the Taskforce on Antimicrobial Resistance (TFAMR) from 2007–2011. In 2016 Governments agreed to re-convene the TFAMR with a broader mandate to address the entire food chain and to report back to the Codex Commission by 2020 [10]. The Terms of Reference are: to revise the *Code of Practice to Minimize and Contain Antimicrobial Resistance* and to develop new *Guidelines on integrated monitoring and surveillance of antimicrobial resistance*.

Gaining consensus agreement through this Codex/TFAMR process may not be easy, particularly as these two documents will also be directly and indirectly endorsing the use of antimicrobials in the food chain. Which antimicrobials can be used in the food chain and in what circumstances represents a highly contested political agenda, particularly antimicrobials used for growth promotion and those deemed essential for human medicine. Codex Guidelines endorsed by Member States may also provide direct or indirect legitimacy for the use of these antimicrobials.

Unlike WTO negotiations, Codex/TFAMR negotiations enable participation and active input from non-government entities. A reading of the open-source negotiating draft documents with input from governments, industry and consumer representatives provide insights into some of the more contentious areas [11]. While few would argue the need for global collaboration (such as the TFAMR process) to minimize the spread of AMR microorganisms is important but if significant differences arise over containing the use of antimicrobials in the food chain this could in-effect serve to hinder government action to proactively protect consumers.

The question of consistency with WTO rules is often a good excuse for government inaction. And an added factor to be cognizant of—given the 'standard setting' role of Codex which links directly into related WTO obligations—is that Codex standards can, and are, often used to justify positions taken in WTO Trade Dispute cases. Or trade disagreements arising when Sanitary and Phytosanitary (SPS) or Technical Barriers to Trade (TBT) agreements are enacted to restrict or place conditionality on imports.

The use of antimicrobials in the food chain is a politically and scientifically contested agenda. And, despite the UN General Assembly 'public health security' framing and political endorsement of the WHO AMR One Health framework and the Global Action Plan (GAP) [12], the Codex/TFAMR parameters open for discussion may not sufficiently prioritize or be consistent with 'human health' priorities. Given that a key human health priority is to maintain the efficacy of medically important antimicrobials, so the veracity of action taken to achieve this will be a significant indicator. AMR policy makers should monitor this agenda closely.

For example, to date, neither of the TFAMR draft negotiation texts refer to the WHO Guidelines on Use of Medically Important Antimicrobials in Food-producing Animals biocides appear to now be excluded; and, altering Codex Maximum Residue Limits (MRL) to consider MRLs for medically important antimicrobials do not seem to be open for discussion.

4. AMR One Health Policies: Role of the World Trade Organization (WTO)

The WTO along with other international agencies has responded to the United Nations General Assembly Resolution on AMR. WTO Director General, Azevedo, has stated the existing WTO framework provides non-discriminatory measures and flexibility for governments to address AMR One Health policies especially around food safety [13]. Azevedo is stating the obvious—it is government's responsibility to activate the legal and regulatory framework to protect their citizens.

AMR in the food chain is a new and complex challenge but implementing such legal and regulatory policies referred to by the WTO DG may not be simply. The international trade environment has expanded considerable since the WTO was established and is more legally complex. National trade policy and the governance framework often have to account for both WTO obligations and broader more intrusive obligations imbedded in new FTAs which may limit the scope for independent national based policy development.

Also, some important structural and capacity issues may be relevant. For example, governments who have lost some in-house regulatory and governance capacity through adopting neo-liberal market based self-regulation strategies and some regulatory limitations flowing from harmonization and trade facilitation policies. Public health experts are often not sufficiently involved in these trade negotiations.

Azevedo's view that the WTO enables implementation of AMR One Health strategies rests on government's commitment at the national level to manage/protect the domestic and export food chain in line with WTO obligations. For food-related imports the Sanitary and Phytosanitary (SPS) or Technical Barriers to Trade (TBT) agreements can be activated but have a relatively narrow interpretive space unless backed up by national regulations.

This WTO report to Codex/TFAMR also records individual governments' input on AMR issues linked to SPS reporting and illustrates some sensitive trade access issues yet to be tested, particularly related to proposed EU regulations [14] (pp. 8–12) The TBT provisions are also likely to be a strong focus as consumers demand of governments more accurate labelling information on antimicrobial use [15].

Implementing longer term SPS measures may rely on specific 'scientific evidence-based data' i.e., directly linking food to human transfer of AMR microorganisms. Emergency measures to contain contaminated food imports are generally considered to be short-term temporary measures. In implementing national regulations that are compliant with WTO obligations the key concept is 'non-discrimination' (in trade parlance—national treatment provisions). This FAO/WTO 'toolkit' is an excellent guide to comprehend these trade rules and obligations for both policy makers and non-WTO experts [16] (pp. 12–17).

5. State of Play: Codex TFAMR Negotiations on AMR in the Food Chain

The health concerns linked to AMR in the food chain encompass both the pathogenic and non-pathogenic AMR microorganisms as both can have serious health consequences [17] (pp. 7–10). It is not yet clear how the 'non-pathogenic' AMR microorganisms in the food chain will be dealt with in the Codex TFAMR process.

Those involved in AMR research, media and consumers may be surprised to know that there are major gaps in monitoring/surveillance and proactive testing for AMR microorganisms in the food chain. Only in 2016 was the draft proposal from the specially convened London Meeting forwarded to Codex and integrated into TFAMR's mandate to develop surveillance guidelines [18] (p. 5). Few if any countries currently systematically test food imports for the presence of AMR microorganisms (whether immediately harmful or not). The rational for lack of action is often circular—based on claims of not enough scientific evidence and/or on the need to first comply with WTO trade obligations [19].

Even in countries with sophisticated governance processes and reliable economic and trade statistics there are considerable gaps in understanding the volume and use made of antimicrobials in animal production and the AMR consequences flowing from this use.

Antimicrobials used in agriculture and aquaculture production are not well understood and even less is known of the effects of AMR in the environment, wildlife, water, or soil etc. [20] Addressing the largely unknown environmental factors, that link to broader forms of AMR contagion has been particularly slow to receive substantive oversight or policy/regulatory focus [17,20,21]. Only some of these aspects may actually be considered in the Codex TFAMR process.

Always in multilateral negotiations, language, and agreed text describing the terms and definitions of the problem areas and the scope of issues, principles, and definitions that can be legitimately addressed are fundamental. And these definitions will impact on the capacity to agree on meaningful outcomes to address the issues at hand.

The formal intergovernmental negotiations remain non-transparent to the broader public and media but the open-source TFAMR working draft texts to revise the AMR Code of Practice (CRD20) [22] and develop new Surveillance Guidelines (CRD18) [23] are available and convey the complexity and political sensitivity of these negotiations. Most useful in providing a sense of negotiations is the formal reporting prepared for the July 2019 Codex Alimentarius Commission, which synthesizes TFAMR outcomes indicating consensus language and points of difference [24]. Several of these outstanding and contested issues will be worked through intersessionally by the two drafting groups led by US and Netherlands and reported to the next TFAMR negotiations in December 2019.

6. Codex/TFAMR Political Sensitivities and Contentious Issues

The current work program of the Codex TFAMR negotiations indicates a considerable amount of work has yet to be undertaken, particularly on the new issues being addressed. It may also be difficult to meet the 2020 deadline. The following three issues are included below as 'Case Studies' for those who wish to delve further into the negotiating dynamics. These Case Studies illustrate some of the complex issues yet to be dealt with and deserve the attention and active engagement by governments, consumers, media and public health experts.

(1) The scope of the 'food chain'—new issues to be included;
(2) Securing antimicrobials of importance for human medicine;
(3) Interpretation attached to evidence—scientific evidence-based versus precautionary principle.

7. Conclusions

The global transition to safeguard antimicrobials is underway but care will have to be taken to ensure that health security is not derailed by narrow interpretations or vested interests. No doubt, particularly at this stage of the negotiations many of the parameters for discussion have ambiguity built-in and while this might placate some concerns there is always the danger these limitations can become in-built into the decisions eventually evolving from the TFAMR [22] (pp. 3–7).

The many but yet little known consequences of AMR in the food chain will emerge as research efforts intensify and unravel the complex AMR effects on the broader ecosystem, including wildlife, water, and soil. Highly dangerous zoonotic diseases are already impacted by AMR affecting large populations so ongoing threats from zoonotic diseases cannot be neatly compartmentalized or insulated from the effects of AMR microorganisms originating from the food chain [25,26].

Information of actual and possible spread of AMR identified in the Expert Report—including to wildlife, insects, and parasites—are yet to be revealed and some but not all aspects will be examined in the TFAMR discussions. This raises questions of which international organization will take responsibility. Infectious and zoonotic disease experts, with their established links to national security frameworks, should obviously have an interest in how this AMR gap will be addressed. These experts should also be actively inputting into the Codex TFAMR negotiations.

Other interesting developments are emerging alongside the Codex/TFAMR negotiations. Leadership on AMR policy is evolving from investors, finance industry and some in the food sectors with potential to be a powerful force for change. Their strategies are now in advance of many government policies and also the current approach being taken in Codex TFAMR negotiations.

And the 73rd UN General Assembly will convene to consider progress made on AMR and the recommendations developed through its Interagency Coordination Group on Antimicrobial Resistance (IACG) [27]. These deliberations should provide a broader overarching model to drive AMR One Health strategies and provide clearer direction to trade-related AMR negotiations such as the Codex TFAMR.

Achieving consensus on a global approach to minimize the spread of AMR is essential but will require significant leadership and incentives to develop the necessary technical capacity to transition away from relying on antimicrobials. But ultimately it is the responsibility of national governments to maintain public confidence in their food chain and to implement governance and regulatory changes needed to address this global health security threat and protect citizens.

Case Study 1. Defining the Scope of AMR in the Food Chain More Broadly

The TFAMR tasked the Codex Secretariat [28] (provided by FAO/WHO) to develop 'scientific advice' on the scope of AMR in the food chain. The FAO/WHO convened an expert meeting and produced this Summary Report on foodborne antimicrobial resistance—Role of environment, crops and biocides [20]. The primary purpose was to synthesize current scientific literature concerning the transmission of AMR from environmental sources—including from water, soil, wildlife, humans, and equipment.

This Expert Group Report, distributed in advance of the meeting, initially was not formally registered on the TFAMR Website [11] but the FAO representative summarized some findings under the item: Scientific Advice to Codex [24], (pp. 1–2): Recording widespread reports of AMR bacteria contamination of foods of plant origin, numerous documented outbreaks of AMR foodborne infections traced to foods of plant origin clearly indicate the potential of these products to transmit AMR microorganisms to human contaminated from multiple sources: water, soil, wildlife, humans, and equipment, and that "Steps should be taken to reduce the likelihood of antimicrobial agents and antimicrobial-resistant bacteria entering the environment from agriculture practices and agricultural food production should be protected from environmental sources of contamination." [24] (p. 1)

Also, reference made to Good Agricultural Practices—to reduce microbial contamination; and, Integrated Pest Management practices to help reduce the need for antimicrobials; on the use of biocides " … there was strong theoretical and laboratory evidence to indicate biocides select for increased resistance to antimicrobials through cross or co-resistance, but empirical evidence is limited" [24] (p. 2). The expert group recommended biocides should be used according to manufacturers' recommendations.

Closing off some issues around biocides the Codex/TFAMR Report now records this agreement: "Antimicrobials used as biocides, including disinfectants, are excluded from the scope of these guidelines" [24] (p. 10).

Some issues raised in the Expert Group Report [20] will be addressed at the next TFAMR meeting in December 2019 and other elements now integrated for further consideration. For example, the draft Code of Conduct definition of 'the food chain' was endorsed by the TFAMR as: *"Production to consumption continuum including, primary production (food producing animals, plants/crops), harvest/slaughter, packing, processing, storage, transport, and retail distribution to the point of consumption"* [22] (p. 4).

Many very sensitive issues, including defining principles are yet to be settled—use of growth promotors and the introduction of government's developing 'national lists' could be usefully developed (but concerns expressed at the potential of such 'lists' to impact trade) [24] (p. 6).

Also worth noting is the WHO/FAO/OIE Report to the TFAMR contains a long list of forthcoming expert meetings to research/analyze outstanding AMR issues including many raised by the Expert Group [20]. But this will be a lengthy process before relevant data and advice will be available [29].

Given the threat to public health of AMR already affecting the food chain and the broader environment, any delay in taking counter-measures to actively protect citizens from such exposure is highly problematic. Especially if reasons for inaction are predicated on the basis that 'evidence' is not available when screening and testing has not been actively pursued by governments or the food industries responsible, or, data is not made transparently available for research.

Case Study 2: Securing Antimicrobials of Importance for Human Medicine—The WHO CIA List

The WHO has already defined the *List of Critically Important Antimicrobials for Human Medicine* (WHO CIA List) [30] which ranks antimicrobials used in human medicine based on two criteria—importance to human health and the likelihood of resistance transmission through the food chain. The WHO also developed and released what could be described as guidance for implementing this CIA List—*The WHO Guidelines on Use of Medically Important Antimicrobials in Food-producing Animals* (WHO Guidelines) [31].

Given the logical progression of these two WHO documents, which essentially provides important implementation guidance to help preserve the antimicrobials most important for human health, but this appears to be a step too far for some countries not yet ready or prepared to take these steps. This resistance was reflected in the Codex/TFAMR documents which excludes any endorsement of these WHO Guidelines. This is an important issue that will not simply disappear, so some background may be useful.

In 2017 after a two year process the WHO Guidelines were released and immediately drew criticism from the U.S. including in this media release from USDA Acting Chief Scientist questioned the legitimacy of the 'evidence' underpinning them as well as the role of the WHO in developing guidelines over subject matter perceived as being the preserve of the Codex and the OIE [32]. This information document from the WHO clarifies the background to the development of the WHO Guidelines and reiterating its role is to protect public health and the antimicrobials important for human medicine. Antibiotics used only in Animals were not included in the WHO Guidelines [33].

Some business-focused media coverage provided this commentary on the politics behind this unusual public criticism of the WHO's mandate to develop such guidance [34]. A later contrary response from some key US Lawmakers on the Codex/TFAMR negotiations regarding the use of 'growth promoters' demonstrated the level of internal contestation that can arise [35].

This difference in opinion over the WHO Guidelines was carried through to Codex TFAMR negotiations with the WHO representative being asked to clarify the 'status' of the WHO CIA List and its Guidelines. A summary of WHO's response is below but the full explanation should be understood as it clearly defines the WHO's mandate to develop these two reports, the governance and operational procedures underpinning them, and the political flexibility accorded to governments [24].

The WHO's statement appears to clarify that both WHO documents have the same status and includes the following points: Both reports are science based, the primary focus is to protect public health and they are not open to negotiations. Their adoption by the World Health Assembly is not required under WHO rules and implementation by Member States is voluntary [24] (p. 2).

With the WHO Guidelines now a source of political contention and questioning the legitimacy of decision making will prove disruptive. But in this important health security agenda questioning the legitimacy of data also has the potential to create a significant fracturing of the global consensus on AMR One Health Policy. Consumer and Health non-government organization's input to TFAMR indicated their full support for the WHO Guidelines.

This dispute over politically endorsing the WHO Guidelines will not be resolved easily or quickly as it signals implementing these WHO Guidelines to preserve the WHO CIA List may be politically problematic or too difficult for some countries.

However, in stark contrast, the recommendations outlined in the OIE List of Antimicrobial Agents of Veterinary Importance [36] and the WHO CIA List [30] are being simultaneously supported. But there are obvious significant compatibility problems that run counter to the objectives of the WHO CIA List. Endorsement of the OIE List sanctions the use of many of the medically important antimicrobials listed in the WHO's CIA List.

The two documents may be individually internally consistent according to the guidance for developing them, but not compatible for delivering the objective of preserving the effectiveness of medically important antimicrobials for human use—the WHO CIA List.

This, of course, is not the only difference in approach, and it would be naïve to expect that such political differences would not arise when significant economic interests are at stake. But questioning the legitimacy of the WHO Guidelines, particularly by such a powerful player as the U.S. could put a break on measures to reduce using medically important antimicrobials that are currently extensively used in food production. Other interested parties may welcome this dispute to delay transitioning away from antimicrobial use. Worth noting, the TFAMR has not yet substantially focused on antimicrobials important for humans also used in crop production or the broader environment [20,37]. These issues will also be highly relevant for zoonotic and infectious disease experts.

Interestingly, asset managers of large investments in the global food industry are moving well ahead of the deliberations in Codex (and many governments). Their agenda links into the WHO CIA list and supports many of the implementation elements contained in the WHO Guidelines [38]. These corporate bodies are aware and expecting AMR trade regulations to be enacted [39] to preserve antimicrobials important for human health. The EU being the most advanced and its One Health Strategy includes commitment to act to protect citizens, food producers and that the efforts made by EU farmers " . . . are not compromised by the non-prudent use of antimicrobials in EU trading partners" [40]. The U.S. FDA Strategy for the Safety of Imported Food also indicates a strategic focus on consumer safety [41].

Case Study 3: The Political Agenda: Scientific-Evidence Based Data versus Precautionary Principle

For a complex subject such as 'AMR in the food chain' the interpretation of what constitutes 'evidence' and the legitimacy this conveys matters—particularly in Codex [42], OIE [43], and the WTO [44] trade-related deliberations. To state the obvious, scientific evidence-based data matters but there are numerous examples of scientific evidence-based claims being overturned as so narrow to be almost meaningless or totally unjustifiable, including many attached to controversial health and food issues i.e. tobacco use, and obesity issues.

AMR also shines a light on the need to implement and develop basic hygiene and public health infrastructure. Developing countries' technical capacity/resources to minimize the dangers of AMR in the food chain are yet to be sufficiently addressed [45]. From an economic and development perspective, those countries relying on export earnings from food production are particularly vulnerable. But for those with well-developed public health systems there remains considerable resistance to transparently collect or test the basic data needed to analyze consequences of antibiotic use in their food producing animals and agriculture.

A reading of the many submissions made into the TFAMR negotiations by government, industry and consumer representatives should leave the reader in no doubt of the underlying sensitivities and interpretations of 'valid' scientific data and risk. Some of these positions may however be overtaken by other events. For example, the WTO Secretariat's Report to the TFAMR demonstrates that multilateral dialogue on trade and AMR in the food chain is being opened up to further scrutiny outside of Codex. WTO Members engaged in a substantive dialogue on AMR issues in the SPS Committee for the first time, primarily focused on EU legislative intentions to address AMR in the food chain [14].

Trop. Med. Infect. Dis. **2019**, *4*, 54

This EU regulatory information provided is important and covers a range of issues and given the response from several countries will be politically sensitive and played out in both Codex and WTO forums. Topics worth noting being developed by the EU include legislative measures: Addressing public health risk of AMR; reserving certain antimicrobials for treatment of infections in humans only; misuse of antimicrobials in medicated feed for prophylaxis and limiting treatment duration. The report records interesting responses and questions to the EU representative from several governments. The report also includes a list of 'regular and emergency' SPS and TBT Notifications submitted by Member States.

The debate opened up in the WTO SPS Committee may not yet have fully registered at the December Codex/TFAMR meeting but is significant. These new inputs now formally expressed to the SPS Committee illustrate further the importance of fully integrating WTO and Codex policy into national AMR One Health strategic planning.

For an observer of the Codex/TFAMR negotiations it is interesting to note that national-based AMR One Health implementation policies are actively reducing human access to antimicrobials. And at the global level, governments have politically endorsed the position that antimicrobials need to be protected and treated as a global public good. Contrasting this, reaching agreement on action to stop or reduce the non-therapeutic use of antimicrobials for food-producing animals and also to preserve medically important antimicrobials for humans, seem to require a much higher standard of scientific evidence-based data. As consumers' understanding of the AMR One Health agenda develops, they may not support such reticence to act on this important health security issue.

Funding: This research received no funding.

Conflicts of Interest: The author declares no conflict of interest.

References

1. United Nations Seventy-First Session of the General Assembly—Political Declaration of the High-Level Meeting on Antimicrobial Resistance, A/RES/71/3 held on 21 September 2016, Resolution Adopted 5 October 2016. Available online: http://www.un.org/en/ga/search/view_doc.asp?symbol=A/RES/71/3 (accessed on 4 February 2019).
2. Review of Antimicrobial Resistance. Available online: https://amr-review.org/ (accessed on 14 February 2019).
3. Burnham, J.P.; Olsen, M.A.; Kollef, M.H. Re-Estimating Annual Deaths Due to Multidrug-Resistant Organism Infections. Available online: https://www.cambridge.org/core/journals/infection-control-and-hospital-epidemiology/article/reestimating-annual-deaths-due-to-multidrugresistant-organism-infections/C9B09A787FCCA1EA992AF45066F3FF7C (accessed on 15 February 2019).
4. CIDRAP. New Estimates Aim to Define the True Burden of Superbug Infections. Available online: http://www.cidrap.umn.edu/news-perspective/2019/02/new-estimates-aim-define-true-burden-superbug-infections (accessed on 14 February 2019).
5. WTO. Overview: The TRIPS Agreement. Available online: https://www.wto.org/english/tratop_e/trips_e/intel2_e.htm (accessed on 10 February 2019).
6. European Union. Understanding EU Reach. Available online: https://echa.europa.eu/regulations/reach/understanding-reach (accessed on 10 February 2019).
7. WTO. Panel Upholds Australia Plain Packaging Policy for Tobacco Products. Available online: https://www.ictsd.org/bridges-news/bridges/news/wto-panel-upholds-australia-plain-packaging-policy-for-tobacco-products (accessed on 10 February 2019).
8. Guardian. Diversion tactics: How Big Pharma is Muddying the Waters on Animal Antibiotics. Available online: https://www.theguardian.com/environment/2018/jun/19/animal-antibiotics-calm-down-about-your-chicken-says-big-pharma (accessed on 5 March 2019).
9. Codex Scorecard. Available online: http://www.fao.org/fao-who-codexalimentarius/thematic-areas/antimicrobial-resistance/en/-c437070 (accessed on 14 February 2019).

10. Ad hoc Codex. Intergovernmental Task Force on Antimicrobial Resistance (TFAMR). Available online: http: //www.fao.org/fao-who-codexalimentarius/committees/committee/en/?committee=TFAMR (accessed on 4 February 2019).

11. Ad Hoc Codex. Intergovernmental Task force on Antimicrobial Resistance—TFAMR 6th Session, 10/12/2018-14/12/2018 Busan, Republic of Korea. Available online: http://www.fao.org/fao-who-codexalimentarius/meetings/detail/en/?meeting=TFAMR&session=6 (accessed on 4 February 2019).

12. WHO. Global Action Plan on Antimicrobial Resistance. Available online: https://www.who.int/antimicrobial-resistance/global-action-plan/en/ (accessed on 5 March 2019).

13. WTO. Director General, Azevêdo. A. Statement to Trilateral meeting with WHO, WIPO and WTO, How WTO. Can Help to Meet Challenge of Antimicrobial Resistance, Geneva, 16 October 2016. Available online: https://www.wto.org/english/news_e/spra_e/spra142_e.htm (accessed on 4 February 2019).

14. Ad Hoc Codex. Intergovernmental Task force on Antimicrobial Resistance: Matters Arising from Other Relevant International Organizations (OECD, World Bank, World Customs Organization, WTO). Available online: http://www.fao.org/fao-who-codexalimentarius/sh-proxy/en/?lnk=1&url=https%3A%2F%2Fworkspace.fao.org%2Fsites%2Fcodex%2FMeetings%2FCX-804-06%2FWD%2Famr06_04e.pdf (accessed on 27 February 2019).

15. ReAct. Antibiotic Footprint: Change the Way Food is Labeled? Available online: https://www.reactgroup.org/news-and-views/news-and-opinions/year-2019/antibiotic-footprint-change-the-way-food-is-labelled/ (accessed on 27 February 2019).

16. The Food and Agriculture Organization of the UN; World Trade Organization. Trade and Food Standards 2017. Available online: http://www.fao.org/3/a-i7407e.pdf (accessed on 4 February 2019).

17. UK Science and Innovation Network. Wellcome Trust and USA CDC. Initiatives for Addressing Antimicrobial Resistance in the Environment. Available online: https://wellcome.ac.uk/sites/default/files/antimicrobial-resistance-environment-report.pdf (accessed on 21 February 2019).

18. Codex. Report of the Physical Working Group on AMR, London December 2016. Available online: http://www.fao.org/fao-who-codexalimentarius/sh-proxy/en/?lnk=1&url=https%253A%252F%252Fworkspace.fao.org%252Fsites%252Fcodex%252FMeetings%252FCX-701-40%252FWD%252Fcac40_12_Add2e.pdf (accessed on 5 March 2019).

19. George, A.; George. Antimicrobial Resistance, Trade, Food Safety and Security. *One Health* **2018**, *5*, 6–8. [CrossRef] [PubMed]

20. FAO; WHO. Expert Meeting on Foodborne Antimicrobial Resistance: Role of Environment, Crop and Biocides. 2018. Available online: https://www.who.int/foodsafety/areas_work/antimicrobial-resistance/FAO_WHO_AMR_Summary_Report_June2018.pdf?ua=1 (accessed on 6 February 2019).

21. Collignon, P.; Beggs, J.J.; Walsh, T.R.; Gandra, S.; Laxminarayan, R. Anthropological and Socioeconomic Factors Contributing to Global Antimicrobial Resistance: A Univariate and Multivariable Analysis. *Lancet Planet. Health* **2018**, *2*, e398–e405. [CrossRef]

22. Codex TFAMR. Proposed Draft Revision of the Code of Practice to Minimize and Contain Foodborne Antibiotic Resistance. Available online: http://www.fao.org/fao-who-codexalimentarius/sh-proxy/en/?lnk=1&url=https%253A%252F%252Fworkspace.fao.org%252Fsites%252Fcodex%252FMeetings%252FCX-804-06%252FCRDs%252Famr6_CRD20x.pdf (accessed on 9 February 2019).

23. Codex TFAMR. Proposed Draft Guidelines on Integrated Monitoring and Surveillance of Foodborne Antimicrobial Resistance. Available online: http://www.fao.org/fao-who-codexalimentarius/sh-proxy/en/?lnk=1&url=https%253A%252F%252Fworkspace.fao.org%252Fsites%252Fcodex%252FMeetings%252FCX-804-06%252FCRDs%252Famr6_CRD18x.pdf (accessed on 9 February 2019).

24. Report of the Sixth Session of the Codex Ad Hoc Intergovernmental Task Force on Antimicrobial Resistance, Busan, Korea, 10–14 December 2018. Available online: http://www.fao.org/fao-who-codexalimentarius/sh-proxy/en/?lnk=1&url=https%253A%252F%252Fworkspace.fao.org%252Fsites%252Fcodex%252FMeetings%252FCX-804-06%252FREPORT%252FFINAL+REPORT%252FREP19_AMRe.pdf (accessed on 24 January 2019).

25. Cantas, L.; Suer, K. Review: The Important Bacterial Zoonoses in "One Health' Concept. Available online: https://www.ncbi.nlm.nih.gov/pmc/articles/PMC4196475/ (accessed on 13 February 2019).

26. European Centre for Disease Prevention and Control (ECDC). Antimicrobial Resistance in Zoonotic Bacteria Still High in Humans, Animals and Food Say ECDC and EFSA. Available online: https://ecdc. europa.eu/sites/portal/files/documents/Pressrelease_ECDCEFSA_AMRzoonoses2016.pdf (accessed on 13 February 2019).

27. Interagency Coordination Group on Antimicrobial Resistance: Draft Recommendations. Available online: https://www.who.int/antimicrobial-resistance/interagency-coordination-group/Draft_IACG_recommendations_for_public_discussion_290119.pdf (accessed on 23 February 2019).

28. Codex Secretariat. Available online: http://www.fao.org/fao-who-codexalimentarius/about-codex/codex-secretariat/en/ (accessed on 20 February 2019).

29. Codex TFAMR. Matters Arising from FAO, WHO and OIE Including The Report of the Joint FAO/WHO Expert Meeting (in Collaboration with OIE) on Foodborne Antimicrobial Resistance. Available online: http://www.fao.org/fao-who-codexalimentarius/sh-proxy/en/?lnk=1&url=https%253A%252F%252Fworkspace.fao.org%252Fsites%252Fcodex%252FMeetings%252FCX-804-06%252FWD%252Famr06_03e.pdf (accessed on 9 February 2019).

30. WHO. List of Critically Important Antimicrobials (WHO CIA List). Available online: https://www.who.int/foodsafety/areas_work/antimicrobial-resistance/cia/en/ (accessed on 10 February 2019).

31. WHO. Guidelines on Use of Medically Important Antimicrobials in Food-Producing Animals. Available online: https://www.who.int/foodsafety/publications/cia_guidelines/en/ (accessed on 8 February 2019).

32. USDA. Chief Scientist Statement on WHO Guidelines on Antibiotics. Available online: https://www. usda.gov/media/press-releases/2017/11/07/usda-chief-scientist-statement-who-guidelines-antibiotics (accessed on 8 February 2019).

33. WHO. Food Safety Antimicrobial Resistance in the Food Chain. Available online: https://www.who.int/foodsafety/areas_work/antimicrobial-resistance/amrfoodchain/en/ (accessed on 20 February 2019).

34. Martin, A.; Hopkins, J.S. *Bloomberg. Trump's USDA Fight Global Guidelines on Livestock Antibiotics*; Bloomberg: New York, NY, USA, 24 July 2018; Available online: https://www.bloomberg.com/news/articles/2018-07-23/trump-s-usda-fights-global-guidelines-on-livestock-antibiotics (accessed on 8 February 2019).

35. Martin, A. Bloomberg, Lawmakers Questions USA > Position on Antimicrobial Use in Livestock 8 December 2018. Available online: https://www.bloomberg.com/news/articles/2018-12-07/lawmakers-question-u-s-position-on-antibiotic-use-in-livestock (accessed on 10 February 2019).

36. OIE. List of Antimicrobial Agents of Veterinary Importance. Available online: http://www.oie.int/fileadmin/Home/eng/Our_scientific_expertise/docs/pdf/AMR/A_OIE_List_antimicrobials_May2018.pdf (accessed on 10 February 2019).

37. Codex TFAMR. Matters Referred by the Codex Alimentarius Commission and other Subsidiary bodies. Available online: http://www.fao.org/fao-who-codexalimentarius/sh-proxy/en/?lnk=1&url=https%253A%252F%252Fworkspace.fao.org%252Fsites%252Fcodex%252FMeetings%252FCX-804-06%252FWD%252Fam06_02e.pdf (accessed on 20 February 2019).

38. FAIRR. Farm Animal Investment Risk and Return: Investor Statement on Antibiotics Stewardship. Available online: https://www.neiinvestments.com/documents/PublicPolicyAndStandards/2017/InvestorStatementonAntibioticsStewardship.pdf (accessed on 8 February 2019).

39. Reducing Agricultural Antibiotics, Can Resistance in Farm Animals be Prevented from Spreading to Humans? Available online: https://www.gbm.hsbc.com/insights/global-research/reducing-agricultural-antibiotics (accessed on 21 February 2019).

40. A European One Health Action Plan Against Antimicrobial Resistance (AMR). Available online: https://ec.europa.eu/health/amr/sites/amr/files/amr_action_plan_2017_en.pdf (accessed on 20 February 2019).

41. USA Food and Drug Administration. (FDA) for the Safety of Imported Food. Available online: https://www.fda.gov/Food/GuidanceRegulation/ImportsExports/Importing/ucm631747.htm (accessed on 27 February 2019).

42. Codex and Science. Available online: http://www.fao.org/fao-who-codexalimentarius/about-codex/science/en/ (accessed on 9 February 2019).

43. OIE Standards and International Trade. Available online: http://www.oie.int/animal-welfare/oie-standards-and-international-trade (accessed on 9 February 2019).

44. WTO Agreements and Public Health. Available online: https://www.wto.org/english/res_e/booksp_e/who_wto_e.pdf (accessed on 9 February 2019).

45. World Bank. Drug-Resistant Infections: A Threat to Our Economic Future (vol2) Final Report. Available online: http://documents.worldbank.org/curated/en/323311493396993758/final-report (accessed on 10 February 2019).

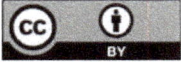

Tropical Medicine and Infectious Disease

MDPI

Review

Policy and Science for Global Health Security: Shaping the Course of International Health

Kavita M. Berger [1,*], James L. N. Wood [2], Bonnie Jenkins [3,4], Jennifer Olsen [5], Stephen S. Morse [6], Louise Gresham [7], J. Jeffrey Root [8], Margaret Rush [1], David Pigott [9,10], Taylor Winkleman [11], Melinda Moore [12,†], Thomas R. Gillespie [13,14], Jennifer B. Nuzzo [15], Barbara A. Han [16], Patricia Olinger [17], William B. Karesh [18], James N. Mills [13], Joseph F. Annelli [19], Jamie Barnabei [20], Daniel Lucey [21] and David T. S. Hayman [22,*]

[1] Gryphon Scientific, LLC, 6930 Carroll Avenue, Suite 810, Takoma Park, MD 20912, USA; margaret@gryphonscientific.com

[2] Disease Dynamics Unit, Department of Veterinary Medicine, University of Cambridge, Madingley Road, Cambridge CB3 0ES, UK; jlnw2@cam.ac.uk

[3] Brookings Institution, 1775 Massachusetts Avenue NW, Washington, DC 20036, USA; bonniedjenkins@gmail.com

[4] Women of Color Advancing Peace, Security and Conflict Transformation, 3695 Ketchum Court, Woodbridge, VA 22193, USA

[5] Rosalynn Carter Institute for Caregiving, Georgia Southwestern State University, 800 GSW State University Drive, Americus, GA 31709, USA; jenolsen.drph@gmail.com

[6] Department of Epidemiology, Mailman School of Public Health, Columbia University, 722 West 168th St., New York, NY 10032, USA; ssm20@cumc.columbia.edu

[7] Ending Pandemics and San Diego State University, San Diego, CA 92182, USA; lgresham@sdsu.edu

[8] U.S. Department of Agriculture, National Wildlife Research Center, Fort Collins, CO 80521, USA; Jeff.Root@aphis.usda.gov

[9] Institute for Health Metrics and Evaluation, Department of Health Metrics Sciences, University of Washington, 2301 Fifth Avenue, Suite 600, Seattle, WA 98121, USA; pigottdm@uw.edu

[10] Wellcome Centre for Human Genetics, Nuffield Department of Medicine, University of Oxford, Roosevelt Drive, Oxford OX3 7BN, UK

[11] Next Generation Global Health Security Network, Washington, DC 20001, USA; t.winkleman.dvm@gmail.com

[12] RAND Corporation, 1200 South Hayes St., Arlington, VA 22202, USA

[13] Population Biology, Ecology, and Evolution Program, Emory University, Atlanta, GA 30322, USA; thomas.gillespie@emory.edu (T.R.G.); wildlifedisease@gmail.com (J.N.M.)

[14] Department of Environmental Health, Rollins School of Public Health, 1518 Clifton Road, Atlanta, GA 30322, USA

[15] Center for Health Security, Johns Hopkins University School of Public Health, Pratt Street, Baltimore, MD 21202, USA; jnuzzo1@jhu.edu

[16] Cary Institute of Ecosystem Studies, Box AB Millbrook, NY 12545, USA; hanb@caryinstitute.org

[17] Environmental, Health and Safety Office (EHSO), Emory University, 1762 Clifton Rd., Suite 1200, Atlanta, GA 30322, USA; patty.olinger@emory.edu

[18] EcoHealth Alliance, 460 West 34th Street, New York, NY 10001, USA; karesh@ecohealthalliance.org

[19] Practical One Health Solutions, LLC, New Market, MD 21774, USA; pohsolutions@gmail.com

[20] Plum Island Animal Disease Center, Department of Homeland Security, Greenport, NY 11944, USA; jbarnabei87@gmail.com

[21] Department of Medicine Infectious Disease, Georgetown University, 600 New Jersey Avenue, NW Washington, DC 20001, USA; daniel.lucey8@gmail.com

[22] EpiLab, Infectious Disease Research Centre, School of Veterinary Science, Massey University, Private Bag, 11 222, Palmerston North 4442, New Zealand

*   Correspondence: kberger@gryphonscientific.com (K.M.B.); d.t.s.hayman@massey.ac.nz (D.T.S.H.); Tel.: +1-240-485-2559 (K.M.B.); +64-06-951-6047 (D.T.S.H.)

†   Deceased, 17 January 2019.

Received: 17 February 2019; Accepted: 8 April 2019; Published: 10 April 2019

Trop. Med. Infect. Dis. **2019**, *4*, 60

Abstract: The global burden of infectious diseases and the increased attention to natural, accidental, and deliberate biological threats has resulted in significant investment in infectious disease research. Translating the results of these studies to inform prevention, detection, and response efforts often can be challenging, especially if prior relationships and communications have not been established with decision-makers. Whatever scientific information is shared with decision-makers before, during, and after public health emergencies is highly dependent on the individuals or organizations who are communicating with policy-makers. This article briefly describes the landscape of stakeholders involved in information-sharing before and during emergencies. We identify critical gaps in translation of scientific expertise and results, and biosafety and biosecurity measures to public health policy and practice with a focus on One Health and zoonotic diseases. Finally, we conclude by exploring ways of improving communication and funding, both of which help to address the identified gaps. By leveraging existing scientific information (from both the natural and social sciences) in the public health decision-making process, large-scale outbreaks may be averted even in low-income countries.

Keywords: One Health; zoonoses; Ebola virus; emerging infectious diseases

---

1. Introduction

For decades, researchers have been studying infectious diseases affecting people, domestic and wild animals, and plants. Researchers have characterized emerging infectious diseases from viruses such as Human Immunodeficiency Virus (HIV) [1] and Severe Acute Respiratory Syndrome (SARS) coronavirus (CoV) [2,3], and bacteria such as *Escherichia coli* O104:H4 in Germany and France [4,5]. Approximately 75% of emerging pathogens have their origins in non-human reservoir hosts and are classic examples of zoonoses [6]. Furthermore, antimicrobial resistance among zoonotic diseases has become a significant health security challenge [7–9]. Combined with vaccine research and development (R&D) and immunization campaigns, scientific studies have contributed to the prevention or reduction of disease transmission globally [10–12]. Existing scientific knowledge and experience could be built upon to prevent or mitigate future outbreaks. However, under pressure to respond quickly to emerging outbreaks, decision-makers struggle to identify effective and relevant medical and non-medical public health response measures because they may not have available information about the causative agents, assessments of potential health and/or economic effects, effective biosafety and infection control measures, information about societally appropriate control measures, and ready risk communication measures for their constituents. Three primary types of gaps (data and models, safety and security, and cultural awareness) limit the translation of research findings in the decision-making process before, during, and after emergencies.

The 2014–2016 West-African Ebola virus disease (EVD) outbreak reinforced the concept that a major pathogen outbreak in one country can affect other countries throughout the region and world, and highlighted the aforementioned gaps in leveraging existing knowledge and practices to facilitate outbreak response [13,14]. This outbreak demonstrated that urban settings, socio-cultural traditions, and local migration affect outbreak dynamics. These lessons, along with the development and use of an experimental Ebola virus vaccine, contributed to very different responses in the 2018 outbreaks in the Democratic Republic of Congo (DRC) [15]. However, conflict and an unsafe public health response environment in the DRC towards the end of 2018 and into 2019 have led to a significant increase of known cases to over 1000 [16]. As long as the security situation ensues, the number of cases will continue to increase and the ability of researchers to collect information about circulating strains will be hampered.

In addition, advancing genomic sequencing capabilities are used to generate increasing amounts of data about bacteria, viruses, and other microorganisms in different locations. For example, the

U.S. government has supported sequencing and modelling studies to identify different strains of pathogens in nature and evaluate their potential to initiate or drive outbreaks of local and international concern. The Canadian government, World Health Organization, U.S. government, non-governmental organizations (e.g., ProMED-mail), private companies, and research groups have leveraged data analytics platforms to analyze these and other available data and attempt to identify potential outbreaks before they become significant public health problems [17–20]. These platforms integrate epidemiological or syndromic data from a variety of sources, both official (e.g., Ministry of Health reports) and unofficial (e.g., media reports) sources, to help identify potential outbreaks as early as possible. The utility of these and related efforts relies on access to data, the sharing of which is governed by different international and national-level policies, and on awareness among policy-makers that scientific information, however uncertain, can inform initial and ongoing assessments of infectious disease risk and response [21,22]. These platforms do not appear to incorporate systematically the results from environmental scanning, modeling, and other related research fields. These platforms vary by the purpose, their intended stakeholders, the data they integrate, their analytic capabilities and methodologies, their accuracy, and other factors, all of which have different utility to public health decision-makers [23–25].

Although these results often are published in academic literature, decision-makers may not be aware that the studies exist, may not have access to the publication or the information contained therein, may not know how best to integrate the information into their decision-making processes, and/or may prefer to rely on scientific studies conducted by government, rather than non-governmental, researchers. Therefore, the existence of research, biosurveillance platforms, and official reporting mechanisms for infectious disease events does not necessarily indicate that these activities intersect and inform each other.

As observed after the launch of the 2014 Global Health Security Agenda (GHSA) and associated action packages, much of the scientific information accessed by human and animal health officials and public health decision-makers was, and continues to be, generated by local and/or central diagnostic laboratories [26–28]. Continuing to address gaps in these capabilities can lead to significant advances in disease prevention, such as a recent response to Nipah virus in India [29]. However, different sectors (specifically, academic, industry, and non-profit organizations) comprise the science and technology communities that develop and provide the tools necessary for detection, characterization, and analysis of infectious disease events. The results of this basic and applied research are published in scientific articles and discussed at scientific conferences, and genetic sequences and other similar information are deposited in databases, many of which exist for various model systems (e.g., plants and animals) and microbes. The scientists who conduct these studies become experts in their fields, often having the skills to help understand the significance of unusual outbreaks with known pathogens and to characterize new pathogens that resemble the ones they study. For example, in 2003, researchers on three continents who studied known respiratory pathogens were able to identify the first member of the coronavirus family causing widespread pneumonia in humans, the SARS-CoV [2,3,30–33]. In addition, researchers who study insects contribute to the scientific knowledge about how mosquitoes and ticks transmit pathogens such as Zika virus and *Borrelia burgdorferi* (the causative agent of Lyme disease), respectively. However, the expertise of the independent researchers (i.e., researchers who are not embedded within public or veterinary health agencies) and the data they produce often are not included in the decision-making process for outbreak response, unless prior relationships exist between the researchers and the public health decision-makers and practitioners.

The disconnect between research investment in human and animal health decision-making about infectious disease outbreaks and translation of data and expertise generated from research in the decision-making process may limit some early detection and response activities needed to prevent and control infectious disease outbreaks. This article describes the current state of scientific input in the public health decision-making process and highlights the different types of organizations involved in communicating scientific information before and during outbreaks. Based on the identified gaps, we consider approaches for promoting communication and trust-building between scientists (both governmental and non-governmental scientists) and policy-makers to ensure that existing data and knowledge can be brought to bear when preparing for, assessing, and responding to infectious disease incidents. Among these approaches, promoting objective, open communication among policy-makers and researchers (from the natural and social sciences) before, during, and after public health emergencies are critical for achieving the goals of the GHSA and related initiatives focused on reducing natural, accidental, and deliberate biological risks, frequently through the lens of One Heath.

2. Science Informing Global Health Security Decision Making

Information Pathways and Decision-Making in Crises

The flow of scientific information into the global health security decision-making process relies on several key factors, including: (a) networks of experts who are familiar to decision-makers and trusted experts in their respective fields; (b) information that is accessible to organizations and individuals involved in public health response; (c) decision-makers' ability to understand and evaluate scientific information; and (d) the use of scientific information by individual(s) responsible for assessing the public health situation and operational decisions. In this paper, we distinguish between scientific information (i.e., data) collected during an outbreak, and information generated by clinical or fundamental research prior to an outbreak and published in publicly-available literature, regardless of whether it is open access or available for a fee. In addition, we group together organizations involved in data generation, whether through research or epidemiological studies, which includes academic, industrial, non-profit, human and animal diagnostic, and government laboratories. We distinguish these scientists from public health decision-makers and practitioners, who play roles in policy-making and/or health response operations. All of these stakeholders are critical to the effective translation of data to public health emergency prevention, detection, and response.

Under non-emergency conditions, scientific and technical information usually is provided to policy and decision-makers of all levels (e.g., health and agricultural agencies, political leaders, and lawmakers) through a variety of means, including white papers, briefings, informal communication, published papers, and scientific conferences [34,35]. However, the flow of scientific information during emergencies is different, often reflecting the immediacy of the situation. The GHSA and International Health Regulations (IHR) provide a defined process, through guidance, for the generation and reporting of public health emergencies of potential international concern. No clear process exists for compiling and evaluating previously published scientific data to inform public health decision-making. Without trusted networks of experts and organizations that communicate scientific information to policy-makers objectively, interest groups which provide information selectively, may be the prevailing voice [36,37]. This situation may result in policy-makers developing trusted relationships with individuals and organizations with biases, which may limit objective and thorough examination of the human, animal, agricultural, or environmental health problem(s). At the same time, many researchers, though not all, do not engage with policy-makers because they do not believe they play a role in policy or decision-making and/or believe that decision-makers may not be willing to listen to their insights. This lack of engagement can limit the quality and objectivity of information being conveyed to decision-makers.

Limitations in effective translation of scientific information under emergency and non-emergency conditions determine its use in decision-making. For example, if information is perceived as partial (i.e., incomplete and/or highly uncertain) or people communicating the information are perceived as biased, decision-makers may question the utility of the data or disregard it completely. Similarly, data inconsistent with beliefs, traditions, or political agendas may be disregarded and/or discredited to maintain cultural and social realities. For example, a number of parents choose to not vaccinate their children for unsubstantiated reasons, including a disbelief in the necessity of the vaccines, perception that vaccines cause infections rather than prevent them, and belief that vaccines may cause autism [38]. Conversely, more complete data sets, more objective communication of the data, and clearer descriptions of the uncertainty of the data and analytic results may engender greater confidence in the information contributing to the decision-making process, especially if communicated effectively and appropriately for the audience.

In emergency situations, when timing and dynamics change, confidence in scientific information and advice is extremely important. Decision-makers frequently do not have time to identify and familiarize themselves with existing scientific information. Consequently, gaps in knowledge may develop, leading to uncertainty about the utility of scientific data. Similarly, uncertainty in known data also may lead decision-makers to question the utility of the scientific data. In addition, the process for sharing information with decision-makers may be cumbersome, inefficient, or nonexistent, all hampering scientifically-informed decision making. Although these limitations exist in non-emergency situations, they are exacerbated in emergencies. Therefore, during emergencies, decision-makers rely more on established relationships with experts for sourcing scientific information, which may include relevant knowledge and expertise (e.g., 2003 SARS-CoV outbreak) or only public health data, ignoring other sources (e.g., 2014–2016 West Africa EVD outbreak).

3. Key Gaps and Impediments to Science-Driven Decision Making

3.1. Data and Models

Incorporating social, natural, computational, and mathematical science analyses, including collection and characterization of specimens [39], into public health decision-making processes may help prevent future outbreaks of infectious diseases [40]. Full integration of information is difficult to achieve because of a lack of cross-pollination of disciplines and sectors [41]. Under-resourced individuals and organizations (including diagnostic and research laboratories, particularly in low-resource countries) may not have the capacity to conduct needed scientific assessments and communicate results to key audiences, which significantly limits the sharing and use of scientific information by researchers, health officials, and decision-makers. In addition, to evaluate the potential risk of emerging outbreaks, researchers and decision-makers must interpret new scientific findings from multidisciplinary studies and modeling data, which may vary in uncertainty based on the availability and veracity of the input data [42]. The relative lack of inter-disciplinary research and data analysis [43,44] in research of public health relevance contributes to these challenges of data interpretation and risk assessment.

Scientific methodologies, such as ecological niche modeling and spatial regression analyses, could contribute to better situational awareness in public health crises [45–48]. Combining these analyses with existing case studies may improve outbreak prediction and prevention (e.g., recent assessments of mosquito vectors for Zika virus in the United States) [49]. These and other types of modeling approaches [50,51] help to identify the information needs for which little data exist by leveraging results from other studies and revealing key knowledge gaps that, if filled, could improve accuracy and reduce the uncertainty of computational models [42,44,52,53]. As data are generated and analytic capabilities improve, uncertainty associated with modeling and data analysis decreases. Therefore, investments in cross-disciplinary research on ecology, wildlife and domestic animals, human health, behavioral sciences, implementation science, and cultural anthropology are essential for understanding how humans interact with their environments and how these interactions facilitate the emergence of previously unknown, wildlife-derived pathogens in the human population [54–58]. Similar trends can be observed with integration of social and biomedical sciences research, where research on behavioral change can inform compliance with medical interventions [59–61]. Communicating these and other data clearly and concisely to public health decision-makers is important for translating research investments to public health practice [62].

3.2. Safety and Security

From a risk management and infection control perspective, data on the capability of nations to respond to emerging or re-emerging infectious disease events are incomplete and the local traditions that inform control measures generally are not integrated into formal public health responses [63–69]. However, these data play a key role in implementing measures that meet the objectives of the 2005 IHR, OIE (World Organization for Animal Health) Standards, and the GHSA objectives and Action Packages (https://ghsagenda.org/). In 2016, a Commission on a Global Health Risk Framework for the Future highlighted the neglected dimension of security in global health [70]. Still, the ability to protect scientists, healthcare providers, the community, and the environment from exposure to pathogens that could harm public health and safety often is overlooked. However, this situation may change through efforts such as the GHSA 2024 Framework [71].

Critical to successful outbreak prevention and management is recognizing the need to identify, test, and employ biosafety and biosecurity measures that are sustainable and adoptable in local conditions, account for local infrastructure, laws, and social structure, and prevent accidental and deliberate release of studied pathogens. Outbreak investigations for Ebola virus, Middle East Respiratory Syndrome coronavirus (MERS-CoV), and SARS-CoV demonstrated the need for locally effective biosafety measures that protect healthcare workers, diagnostic laboratory workers, and animal health workers from exposure to the outbreak viruses, and biosecurity measures that prevent access to pathogens by malicious actors. Applied research may identify measures that enhance current risk management efforts, such as laboratory and clinical biosafety, biosecurity, and biorisk management.

3.3. Cultural Awareness

Social science research can provide a better understanding of local culture and traditions, which strongly influence pathogen transmission and acceptance of medical and public health interventions [43]. During the 2014–2016 West African EVD outbreak, a lack of cultural awareness about local end-of-life traditions led to ineffective or unintentionally dangerous public health interactions and undocumented infections [72–74]. Eventually, the public health community began identifying approaches to communicate the risk of virus transmission from touching infected bodies, mitigate transmission events through culturally acceptable means, and reduce fear of death through appropriately chosen infection control methods (e.g., use of white, instead of black, body bags in West Africa [75]). Early engagement with communities and social scientists who study the culture, tradition, and linguistics of people from affected areas would help inform communication by decision-makers, mitigation strategies used by public health responders, and trust-building with the local population. Furthermore, leveraging the knowledge gained from these social science disciplines could enhance efforts to build trust among affected individuals rather than allow the persistence of distrust between local communities and foreign health workers [76,77]. Similar approaches should be used towards domestic and wild animal research, with animal and conservation ethics and local cultural and traditions considered.

Research involving bioethics and social equity helps scientists incorporate ethical principles in the design and conduct studies involving human participants affected by public health emergencies [78]. Such studies are critically important for research examining the effectiveness of candidate vaccines and medicines, understanding pathogen transmission and infection in natural settings, and testing non-pharmaceutical interventions for disease prevention and mitigation. Although such studies have been conducted for years, the U.S. National Academies of Science, Engineering, and Medicine highlighted research needs for preparedness and response to public health emergencies and associated bioethical considerations [79]. This focus on the bioethics of disaster research has prompted non-governmental and governmental organizations alike to evaluate challenges and identify solutions to promote ethical practices in research during public health emergencies. Building on this and other social science research can promote the development and implementation of clinical and public health research that takes into account the culture, society, and benefits to and needs of research participants.

4. Potential Solutions

The purpose of much of infectious disease research is to identify pharmaceutical and non-pharmaceutical approaches for preventing, detecting and monitoring, and responding to public health outbreaks of national, regional, and international concern. Data that could inform prevention, detection, and response activities are generated by several different types of studies, including mathematical modeling, epidemiological studies, environmental scanning, life-sciences studies (e.g., microbial genomics), and cultural anthropology. By integrating known, published data in these fields, considering key knowledge gaps and existing areas of uncertainty, scientists can assist public health responders and decision-makers in understanding initial cases and feasible infection control measures. However, the results of these investments have limited utility if they are not being conveyed to policy-makers before the occurrence of and during an emergency. Without this information, human and animal health officials and health care professionals are left to diagnose emerging outbreaks using sub-optimal approaches and driving response efforts that might be unnecessarily ineffective and promulgating distrust in health response efforts.

Three approaches for addressing these gaps are communication, funding, and translation efforts. Although not explicitly described in this paper, international and national policies on data access and decisions made for political or national security purposes present additional challenges to fully informed decision-making. Some of the solutions described in this section may help reduce, but not eliminate, these challenges, highlighting the realities inherent in global governance of public health preparedness and response. Nevertheless, the proposed solutions could improve communication between researchers and decision-makers and enhance translation of research investments to inform public health practice before, during, and after emergencies.

4.1. Communication

Communication strategies that include better articulation and dissemination of existing scientific knowledge and modeling approaches (including their use, gaps, and limitations), their relevance to public health emergencies, and the inherent uncertainties in scientific assessment greatly would enhance high-level public health decision-making before, during, and after emergencies [34]. Better awareness about the types of public health decisions, associated information needs, operational constraints, time pressures of decision-makers, and limitations of current scientific knowledge would enable researchers to communicate scientific information more effectively. Understanding what is required of data and how data are best communicated in public health emergencies would provide researchers with the necessary operational context in which decision-makers must evaluate and base their decisions. With greater appreciation for the limitations of and information needs during the decision-making process, researchers can identify, integrate and distill data of greatest relevance to the specific emergency.

Effective communication can be achieved through active interaction or written documents, and fostered in a variety of venues, including scientific conferences, science and society workshops, and governmental meetings. Although some of these efforts currently are used, their effectiveness can be improved by tailoring communication to the audience. Interactions cultivated among stakeholders before emergencies could promote the development of trusted relationships between decision-makers and scientists, which can serve as the foundation for reach-back during public health emergencies. In addition, interactions through networks, such as the GHSA and associated groups, could promote open lines of communication between governmental health security officials and scientists, facilitating information-sharing and enabling greater understanding of key questions with which decision-makers struggle [35]. These interactions are most effective if they are in place before crises occur and maintained after an emergency ends, which can lead to greater trust and familiarity between policy-makers and researchers and more opportunities for information-sharing in non-emergency situations. Throughout, promoting diversity of scientific expertise and experiences within these communications networks is critical for ensuring that policy-makers receive unbiased, objective information upon which to base their decisions.

4.2. Funding and Open Access

Research investments can enhance detection, characterization, assessment, and response to infectious diseases. However, several challenges exist with the current approaches: (1) limited funding is available for basic research for a majority of infectious diseases, particularly neglected tropical diseases and wildlife-associated, epizootic (animal only) diseases; (2) limited funding opportunities exist for multi-disciplinary, multi-sectoral research and education; (3) limited support is provided for social science research that is relevant to prevention and mitigation of infectious disease outbreaks; (4) research funding continuously changes for many infectious diseases, limiting the sustainability of individual efforts (e.g., the 2018 U.S. President's proposed budget included funding cuts for efforts to prevent and respond to EVD outbreaks even as the 2018 outbreak in the DRC emerged [80,81]); (5) lack of communication from scientists to non-technical audiences, including policy-makers; and (6) lack of evaluation metrics for assessing the effectiveness of scientific input into the public health process.

To counter these challenges, government agencies, intergovernmental organizations, private funders, and philanthropic organizations should develop forward-looking, longer-term initiatives that support basic and applied research in a variety of natural and social sciences, and in efforts promoting integration and translation of scientific data to public health emergency prevention, detection, and response. Although not routinely done, proactive and stable funding for these and other scientific inquiries provides opportunities to increase the knowledge-base from which decision-makers can draw when considering appropriate infection control actions, a suggestion supported by several scientific organizations. For example, longer-term studies, such as those on New World hantaviruses, have produced a great deal of information relevant to public health [82], including changing infection prevalence with species richness [83], the preponderance of infected males [84], and the role of climatic changes in causing fluctuations in rodent reservoir populations and their links to localized, sporadic disease outbreaks. Although these studies were initiated as part of a reactive response to an acute outbreak—in this case, hantavirus pulmonary syndrome—in 1993–1994, the information produced addresses key knowledge gaps that can inform future outbreaks. Similarly, research supported during and after EVD outbreaks has generated data on wildlife reservoir hosts and people's perceptions of health and healthcare practices, both of which could inform future outbreak assessments and response efforts. In addition, funders should establish a process through which the results and assessments can be communicated to public health decision-makers, leveraging the recent movement towards open access publication requirements. As a positive example, the Bill and Melinda Gates Foundation and The Wellcome Trust require all grantees to make their results publicly available, enabling access to various stakeholders, including decision-makers [85–87]. However, access to information does not ensure their use by decision-makers. In addition, new data protection laws may counteract these open access policies of funders and journals [88].

Specific approaches for promoting greater translation of research include scientific staff support for decision-makers, fellowship opportunities, cross-disciplinary cooperation, and strategic funding mechanisms (e.g., contracts and cooperative agreements). Scientists and funders should identify and support the integration and translation of science from multiple sectors, fields, and disciplines to identify key information gaps for global health security and provide the scientific foundation for assessing infectious disease risks. Funding support for training and fellowships can promote explicit scientific input into decision-making and encourage open sharing of data with other researchers and health officials. Researchers and research institutions should aim to shift the culture of data sharing by promoting the open sharing of data with public health practitioners as an academic product on par with publications, decreasing the potential for politicization or biased use of data [70]. Data sharing has been raised with H5N1 influenza A virus, Ebola virus, and Zika virus [89], and informed by efforts to promote equitable benefit of results from the sharing of data and samples from emerging outbreaks [90,91]. In 2014, the U.S. government passed the DATA (Data Transparency and Accountability) Act, which requires that data from federally-funded efforts be made open and available. The U.S. government's DATA.gov website (https://www.data.gov/) is the platform that was developed to store and provide access to the datasets. In addition, agencies such as U.S. Geological Survey now have an 'eternal data' archive called Science Base (https://www.sciencebase.gov/catalog/). Despite these efforts, national policies restricting data access and sharing to foreign entities present new challenges to equitable and reciprocal data sharing, especially as biological research increasingly relies on data science approaches [92].

Approaches for improving communication between researchers and policy-makers, the funding landscape, and open access policies could help promote research that addresses key knowledge gaps in health security policy and practice, and translate funded research to global health decision-making.

4.3. Translation of Data

Looking forward, the 2024 Framework of the Global Health Security Agenda stresses communication, political and financial advocacy, and engagement of a more diverse set of stakeholders [71]. In part, these efforts intend to increase national-level investment and support for addressing shortcomings in human and animal health capabilities that currently limit effective prevention, detection, and response to public health emergencies of international concern. However, the new structure developed to progress towards these GHSA efforts could be enhanced further by including the research community as a critical stakeholder and focusing attention on data sharing among the research, public health, veterinary health, agriculture, and environmental health communities. Active engagement of the scientific arms of research and diagnostic entities (regardless of their sector, whether academic, industry, or government laboratories) with local and national public and veterinary health entities could enable better translation of scientific information to address public health needs. Recent calls for integrating veterinary and human health research to improve One Health efforts, including policy development and implementation, have been published [93,94]. Training on and implementation of data translation, improved strategies for communicating data and their associated limitations and/or statistical significance, and active participation of the scientific community in public health decision-making processes could reveal opportunities for leveraging data in an informative and timely manner.

5. Conclusions

The global burden of infectious diseases and the increased attention to natural, accidental, and deliberate biological threats has resulted in scientific and financial investment in infectious disease research. However, the results of these studies often are not translated to prevention, detection, and response efforts. Furthermore, the needs, receptivity, and stakeholders involved in sharing scientific data before and during emergencies differ, which can lead to barriers towards research translation to human and animal health practice. Overcoming these barriers is necessary to prevent and mitigate emerging and re-emerging infectious diseases, including the recent epidemics caused by Zika virus in the Americas, Yellow fever virus (YFV) in Angola and the DRC, and Ebola virus in the DRC. The public health burden caused by influenza virus has led to the creation of WHO collaborating centers through which data on naturally circulating strains and results from basic and applied research are shared, informing influenza surveillance efforts. In addition, scientific data associated with the Zika virus disease outbreak has been placed in the public domain to facilitate prevention and control of the outbreak. However, these data sharing efforts are inconsistent across outbreaks, as demonstrated by the lack of similar data sharing practice in the YFV outbreak in Africa [95]. Furthermore, sharing of data is not the same as effective communication of the data.

Despite the increased investment for infectious disease research, significant knowledge gaps remain in host–pathogen interactions, urbanization and climactic influences on pathogen transmission, pathogen evolution, interactions between wild and domestic animals and humans, existence of

Trop. Med. Infect. Dis. **2019**, *4*, 60

unknown but naturally occurring pathogens, and other areas of interest. These knowledge gaps introduce uncertainty about what can be concluded from available data, which in turn can raise doubt in the utility of research results and validity of science-based conclusions during decision-making, especially in emergency situations. Advanced engagement and communication between researchers and policy-makers could help identify critical knowledge gaps that could reduce uncertainty levels and promote better trust between scientists and decision-makers. Encouraging and training scientists to recognize and translate research findings to public health decision-makers enhances these efforts. Effective communication and long-term funding are important for providing decision-makers with a clear understanding of what is known and what needs to be determined to improve prevention, detection, and response efforts of current and future outbreaks.

Author Contributions: Conceptualization, all authors; Writing—Original Draft preparation, K.M.B. and D.T.S.H.; Writing—Review and Editing, all authors.

Funding: DTSH is funded by Royal Society Te Apārangi, grant number MAU1701 and MAU1503. SSM is funded by the Arts and Letters Foundation.

Acknowledgments: The driver for this paper and its broad authorship was a workshop held in June 2015, titled "Joint RAPIDD-GHSA Workshop: Policy Implications of Detecting Hemorrhagic Fever Viruses in Wildlife and Domestic Animals". The workshop was held under the auspices of the National Institutes of Health and Department of Homeland Security-funded Research and Policy for Infectious Disease Dynamics (RAPIDD) program and in coordination with the U.S. Department of State. We thank Audrey Thevenon (National Academy of Sciences, Engineering, and Medicine), Rocco Casagrande (Gryphon Scientific), Christopher Hofmann (U.S. Department of State), Ellis McKenzie (National Institutes of Health, sadly deceased), and Bryan Grenfell (Princeton University) for their support.

References

1. Barré-Sinoussi, F.; Chermann, J.-C.; Rey, F.; Nugeyre, M.T.; Chamaret, S.; Gruest, J.; Dauguet, C.; Axler-Blin, C.; Vézinet-Brun, F.; Rouzioux, C. Isolation of a T-lymphotropic retrovirus from a patient at risk for acquired immune deficiency syndrome (AIDS). *Science* **1983**, *220*, 868–871. [CrossRef]

2. Rota, P.A.; Oberste, M.S.; Monroe, S.S.; Nix, W.A.; Campagnoli, R.; Icenogle, J.P.; Peñaranda, S.; Bankamp, B.; Maher, K.; Chen, M.-H.; et al. Characterization of a novel coronavirus associated with severe acute respiratory syndrome. *Science* **2003**, *300*, 1394–1399. [CrossRef] [PubMed]

3. Peiris, J.S.M.; Lai, S.T.; Poon, L.L.M.; Guan, Y.; Yam, L.Y.C.; Lim, W.; Nicholls, J.; Yee, W.K.S.; Yan, W.W.; Cheung, M.T.; et al. Coronavirus as a possible cause of severe acute respiratory syndrome. *Lancet* **2003**, *361*, 1319–1325. [CrossRef]

4. Rohde, H.; Qin, J.; Cui, Y.; Li, D.; Loman, N.J.; Hentschke, M.; Chen, W.; Pu, F.; Peng, Y.; Li, J.; et al. Open-source genomic analysis of shiga-toxin–producing *E. coli* O104:H4. *N. Engl. J. Med.* **2011**, *365*, 718–724. [CrossRef]

5. Frank, C.; Faber, M.; Askar, M.; Bernard, H.; Fruth, A.; Gilsdorf, A.; Höhle, M.; Karch, H.; Krause, G.; Prager, R. Large and ongoing outbreak of haemolytic uraemic syndrome. *Euro Surveill.* **2011**, *16*, 19878. [PubMed]

6. Taylor, L.H.; Latham, S.M.; Woolhouse, M.E. Risk factors for human disease emergence. *Philos. Trans. R. Soc. Lond. Ser. B Biol. Sci.* **2001**, *356*, 983–989. [CrossRef]

7. World Health Organization. Antimicrobial Resistance. Available online: https://www.who.int/en/news-room/fact-sheets/detail/antimicrobial-resistance (accessed on 31 March 2019).

8. Asokan, G.V.; Kasimanickam, R.K. Emerging infectious diseases, antimicrobial resistance and millennium development goals: Resolving the challenges through one health. *Cen. Asian J. Glob. Health* **2013**, *2*, 76. [CrossRef]

9. European Centre for Disease Prevention and Control. Zoonoses: Antimicrobial Resistance Shows no Signs of Slowing Down. Available online: https://ecdc.europa.eu/en/news-events/zoonoses-antimicrobial-resistance-shows-no-signs-slowing-down (accessed on 31 March 2019).
10. Greenwood, B. The contribution of vaccination to global health: Past, present and future. *Philos. Trans. R. Soc. Lond. B Biol. Sci.* **2014**, *369*, 20130433. [CrossRef]
11. Francis, D.P. Success and failures: Worldwide vaccine development and application. *Biologicals* **2010**, *38*, 523–528. [CrossRef]
12. Greenwood, B.; Salisbury, D.; Hill, A.V.S. Vaccines and global health. *Philos. Trans. R. Soc. Lond. B Biol. Sci.* **2011**, *366*, 2733–2742. [CrossRef] [PubMed]
13. Heymann, D.L.; Chen, L.; Takemi, K.; Fidler, D.P. Global health security: The wider lessons from the West African Ebola virus disease epidemic. *Lancet* **2015**, *385*, 1884–1901. [CrossRef]
14. Backer, J.A.; Wallinga, J. Spatiotemporal analysis of the 2014 Ebola epidemic in West Africa. *PLoS Comput. Biol.* **2016**, *12*, e1005210. [CrossRef]
15. World Health Organization. Ebola Vaccine Provides Protection and Hope for High-Risk Communities in the Democratic Republic of the Congo. Available online: http://www.who.int/news-room/feature-stories/detail/ebola-vaccine-provides-protection-and-hope-for-high-risk-communities-in-the-democratic-republic-of-the-congo (accessed on 14 August 2018).
16. Centers for Disease Control and Prevention. Ebola Outbreak in Eastern Democratic Republic of Congo tops 1000 cases. Available online: https://www.cdc.gov/media/releases/2019/s0322-ebola-congo.html (accessed on 31 March 2019).
17. Pellerin, C. DTRA Scientists Develop Cloud-Based Biosurveillance Ecosystem. Available online: https://dod.defense.gov/News/Article/Article/681832/dtra-scientists-develop-cloud-based-biosurveillance-ecosystem/ (accessed on 17 March 2019).
18. Public Health Agency of Canada. About GPHIN. Available online: https://gphin.canada.ca/cepr/aboutgphin-rmispenbref.jsp?language=en_CA (accessed on 14 August 2018).
19. World Health Organization. Global Outbreak Alert and Response Network (GOARN). Available online: http://www.who.int/ihr/alert_and_response/outbreak-network/en/ (accessed on 14 August 2018).
20. ProMED. International Society for Infectious Diseases. Available online: http://www.promedmail.org/ (accessed on 14 February 2019).
21. Holmes, E.C.; Rambaut, A.; Andersen, K.G. Pandemics: spend on surveillance, not prediction. *Nature* **2018**, *558*, 180–182. [CrossRef]
22. Rivers, C.; Scarpino, S. Modelling the trajectory of disease outbreaks works. *Nature* **2018**, *559*, 477. [CrossRef]
23. Milinovich, G.J.; Soares Magalhaes, R.J.; Hu, W. Role of big data in the early detection of Ebola and other emerging infectious disease. *Lancet Glob. Health* **2015**, *3*, PE20–PE21. [CrossRef]
24. Lazer, D.; Kennedy, R.; King, G.; Vespignani, A. The parable of google flu: Traps in big data analysis. *Science* **2014**, *343*, 1203–1205. [CrossRef]
25. Dion, M.; AbdelMalik, P.; Mawudeku, A. Big data and the global public health intelligence network (GPHIN). *Can. Commun. Dis. Rep.* **2015**, *41*, 209–214. [CrossRef]
26. Kennedy, E.D.; Morgan, J.; Knight, N.W. Global health security implementation: Expanding the evidence base. *Health Security* **2018**. [CrossRef]
27. Edelson, M.; Lee, L.M.; Herten-Crabb, A.; Heymann, D.L.; Harper, D.R. Strengthening global public health surveillance through data and benefit sharing. *Emerg. Infect. Dis.* **2018**, *24*, 1324–1330. [CrossRef]
28. Rodier, G.; Greenspan, A.L.; Hughes, J.M.; Haymann, D.L. Global public health security. *Emerg. Infect. Dis.* **2007**, *13*, 1447–1452. [CrossRef]
29. Sadanadan, R.; Arunkumar, G.; Laserson, K.F.; Heretik, K.H.; Singh, S.; Mourya, D.T.; Gangakhedkar, R.R.; Gupta, N.; Sharma, R.; Dhuria, M. Towards global health security: Response to the May 2018 Nipah virus outbreak linked to pteropus bats in Kerala, India. *BMJ Glob. Health* **2018**, *3*, e001086. [CrossRef]
30. Fouchier, R.A.M.; Kuiken, T.; Schutten, M.; van Amerongen, G.; van Doornum, G.J.J.; van den Hoogen, B.G.; Peiris, M.; Lim, W.; Stöhr, K.; Osterhaus, A.D.M.E. Koch's postulates fulfilled for SARS virus. *Nature* **2003**, *423*, 240. [CrossRef]
31. Drosten, C.; Günther, S.; Preiser, W.; Van Der Werf, S.; Brodt, H.-R.; Becker, S.; Rabenau, H.; Panning, M.; Kolesnikova, L.; Fouchier, R.A. Identification of a novel coronavirus in patients with severe acute respiratory syndrome. *N. Eng. J. Med.* **2003**, *348*, 1967–1976. [CrossRef]

32. Falsey, A.R.; Walsh, E.E. Novel coronavirus and severe acute respiratory syndrome. *Lancet* **2003**, *361*, 1312–1313. [CrossRef]

33. Ksiazek, T.G.; Erdman, D.; Goldsmith, C.S.; Zaki, S.R.; Peret, T.; Emery, S.; Tong, S.; Urbani, C.; Comer, J.A.; Lim, W. A novel coronavirus associated with severe acute respiratory syndrome. *N. Eng. J. Med.* **2003**, *348*, 1953–1966. [CrossRef]

34. Whitty, C.J. What makes an academic paper useful for health policy? *BMC Med.* **2015**, *13*, 1. [CrossRef]

35. Cook, C.N.; Mascia, M.B.; Schwartz, M.W.; Possingham, H.P.; Fuller, R.A. Achieving conservation science that bridges the knowledge–action boundary. *Conserv. Biol.* **2013**, *27*, 669–678. [CrossRef]

36. Contandriopoulos, D.; Brousselle, A.; Brenton, M.; Larouche, C.; Champagne, G.; Rivard, G. Policy-making: polarization and interest group influence: Damien Contradriopoulos. *Eur. J. Public Health* **2017**, *27* (Suppl. 3). [CrossRef]

37. Kushel, M.; Bindman, A.B. Healthcare lobbying: Time to make patients the special interest. *Am. J. Med.* **2004**, *116*, 496–497. [CrossRef]

38. World Health Organization. Global Vaccine Safety. Available online: https://www.who.int/vaccine_safety/ initiative/detection/immunization_misconceptions/en/ (accessed on 8 February 2018).

39. DiEuliis, D.; Johnson, K.R.; Morse, S.S.; Schindel, D.E. Opinion: Specimen collections should have a much bigger role in infectious disease research and response. *Proc. Natl. Acad. Sci. USA* **2016**, *113*, 4–7. [CrossRef]

40. Morse, S.S.; Mazet, J.A.; Woolhouse, M.; Parrish, C.R.; Carroll, D.; Karesh, W.B.; Zambrana-Torrelio, C.; Lipkin, W.I.; Daszak, P. Prediction and prevention of the next pandemic zoonosis. *Lancet* **2012**, *380*, 1956–1965. [CrossRef]

41. Manlove, K.R.; Walker, J.G.; Craft, M.E.; Huyvaert, K.P.; Joseph, M.B.; Miller, R.S.; Nol, P.; Patyk, K.A.; O'Brien, D.; Walsh, D.P. "One Health" or three? Publication silos among the one health disciplines. *PLoS Biol.* **2016**, *14*, e1002448. [CrossRef]

42. Chretien, J.-P.; Riley, S.; George, D.B. Mathematical modeling of the West Africa Ebola epidemic. *eLife* **2015**, *4*, e09186. [CrossRef]

43. Wood, J.L.; Leach, M.; Waldman, L.; Macgregor, H.; Fooks, A.R.; Jones, K.E.; Restif, O.; Dechmann, D.; Hayman, D.T.; Baker, K.S.; et al. A framework for the study of zoonotic disease emergence and its drivers: Spillover of bat pathogens as a case study. *Philos. Trans. R. Soc. Lond. Ser. B Biol. Sci.* **2012**, *367*, 2881–2892. [CrossRef]

44. Restif, O.; Hayman, D.T.; Pulliam, J.R.; Plowright, R.K.; George, D.B.; Luis, A.D.; Cunningham, A.A.; Bowen, R.A.; Fooks, A.R.; O'Shea, T.J. Model-guided fieldwork: practical guidelines for multidisciplinary research on wildlife ecological and epidemiological dynamics. *Ecol. Lett.* **2012**, *15*, 1083–1094. [CrossRef]

45. Brierley, L.; Vonhof, M.J.; Olival, K.J.; Daszak, P.; Jones, K.E. Quantifying global drivers of zoonotic bat viruses: A process-based perspective. *Am. Nat.* **2016**, *187*, E53–E64. [CrossRef]

46. Pigott, D.M.; Golding, N.; Mylne, A.; Huang, Z.; Henry, A.J.; Weiss, D.J.; Brady, O.J.; Kraemer, M.U.; Smith, D.L.; Moyes, C.L. Mapping the zoonotic niche of Ebola virus disease in Africa. *eLife* **2014**, *3*, e04395. [CrossRef]

47. Pigott, D.M.; Golding, N.; Mylne, A.; Huang, Z.; Weiss, D.J.; Brady, O.J.; Kraemer, M.U.; Hay, S.I. Mapping the zoonotic niche of Marburg virus disease in Africa. *Trans. R. Soc. Trop. Med. Hyg.* **2015**, *109*, 366–378. [CrossRef]

48. Peterson, A.; Bauer, J.; Mills, J. Ecologic and geographic distribution of filovirus disease. *Emerg. Infect. Dis.* **2004**, *10*, 40–47. [CrossRef]

49. Monaghan, A.J.; Morin, C.W.; Steinhoff, D.F.; Wilhelmi, O.; Hayden, M.; Quattrochi, D.A.; Reiskind, M.; Lloyd, A.L.; Smith, K.; Schmidt, C.A. On the seasonal occurrence and abundance of the Zika virus vector mosquito *Aedes aegypti* in the contiguous United States. *PLoS Curr.* **2016**, *8*. [CrossRef]

50. Han, B.A.; Schmidt, J.P.; Alexander, L.; Bowden, S.E.; Hayman, D.T.S.; Drake, J.M. Undiscovered bat hosts of filoviruses. *PLoS Negl. Trop. Dis.* **2016**, *10*, e0004815. [CrossRef]

51. Hayman, D.T. Biannual birth pulses allow filoviruses to persist in bat populations. *Proc. R. Soc. Lond. B Biol. Sci.* **2015**, *282*, 20142591. [CrossRef]

52. King, A.A.; de Cellès, M.D.; Magpantay, F.M.; Rohani, P. Avoidable errors in the modelling of outbreaks of emerging pathogens, with special reference to Ebola. *Proc. R. Soc. Lond. B Biol. Sci.* **2015**, *282*, 20150347. [CrossRef]

53. Plowright, R.K.; Eby, P.; Hudson, P.J.; Smith, I.L.; Westcott, D.; Bryden, W.L.; Middleton, D.; Reid, P.A.; McFarlane, R.A.; Martin, G. Ecological dynamics of emerging bat virus spillover. *Proc. R. Soc. Lond. B Biol. Sci.* **2015**, *282*, 20142124. [CrossRef]

54. Calvignac-Spencer, S.; Leendertz, S.; Gillespie, T.; Leendertz, F. Wild great apes as sentinels and sources of infectious disease. *Clin. Microbiol. Infect.* **2012**, *18*, 521–527. [CrossRef]

55. Gillespie, T.R.; Nunn, C.L.; Leendertz, F.H. Integrative approaches to the study of primate infectious disease: Implications for biodiversity conservation and global health. *Am. J. Phys. Anthropol.* **2008**, *137*, 53–69. [CrossRef]

56. Anti, P.; Owusu, M.; Agbenyega, O.; Annan, A.; Badu, E.K.; Nkrumah, E.E.; Tschapka, M.; Oppong, S.; Adu-Sarkodie, Y.; Drosten, C. Human-bat interactions in rural West Africa. *Emerg. Infect. Dis.* **2015**, *21*, 1418–1421. [CrossRef]

57. Kamins, A.O.; Restif, O.; Ntiamoa-Baidu, Y.; Suu-Ire, R.; Hayman, D.T.; Cunningham, A.A.; Wood, J.L.; Rowcliffe, J.M. Uncovering the fruit bat bushmeat commodity chain and the true extent of fruit bat hunting in Ghana, West Africa. *Biol. Conserv.* **2011**, *144*, 3000–3008. [CrossRef]

58. Kamins, A.O.; Rowcliffe, J.M.; Ntiamoa-Baidu, Y.; Cunningham, A.A.; Wood, J.L.; Restif, O. Characteristics and risk perceptions of Ghanaians potentially exposed to bat-borne zoonoses through bushmeat. *EcoHealth* **2014**, *12*, 104–120. [CrossRef]

59. Kippax, S. Understanding and integrating the structural and biomedical determinants of HIV infection: A way forward for prevention. *Curr. Opin. HIV AIDS* **2008**, *3*, 489–494. [CrossRef]

60. Mabry, P.L.; Olster, D.H.; Morgan, G.D.; Abrams, D.B. Interdisciplinarity and systems science to improve population health: A view from the NIH office of behavioral and social sciences research. *Am. J. Prev. Med.* **2008**, *35*, S211–S224. [CrossRef]

61. Jin, J.; Sklar, G.E.; Oh, V.M.S.; Li, S.C. Factors affecting therapeutic compliance: A review from the patient's perspective. *Ther. Clin. Risk Manag.* **2008**, *4*, 269.

62. Ogilvie, D.; Craig, P.; Griffin, S.; Macintyre, S.; Wareham, N.J. A translational framework for public health research. *BMC Public Health* **2009**, *9*, 116. [CrossRef]

63. Jephcott, F.L.; Wood, J.L.; Cunningham, A.A. Facility-based surveillance for emerging infectious diseases; diagnostic practices in rural West African hospital settings: Observations from Ghana. *Phil. Trans. R. Soc. B* **2017**, *372*, 20160544. [CrossRef]

64. Manguvo, A.; Mafuvadze, B. The impact of traditional and religious practices on the spread of Ebola in West Africa: Time for a strategic shift. *Pan. Afr. Med. J.* **2015**, *22* (Suppl. 1), 9.

65. Carrion Martin, A.I.; Derrough, T.; Honomou, P.; Kolie, N.; Diallo, B.; Kone, M.; Rodier, G.; Kpoghomou, C.; Jansa, J.M. Social and cultural factors behind community resistance during an Ebola outbreak in a village of the Guinean Forest region, February 2015: A field experience. *Int. Health* **2016**, *8*, 227–229. [CrossRef]

66. Ulin, P.R. African women and AIDS: Negotiating behavioral change. *Soc. Sci. Med.* **1992**, *34*, 63–73. [CrossRef]

67. De Bruym, M. Women and aids in developing countries: The XIIth international conference on the social sciences and medicine. *Soc. Sci. Med.* **1992**, *34*, 249–262. [CrossRef]

68. Ventura-Garcia, L.; Roura, M.; Rell, C.; Posada, E.; Gascon, J.; Aldasoro, E.; Munoz, J.; Pool, R. Socio-cultural aspects of chagas disease: A systematic review of qualitative research. *PLoS Negl. Trop. Dis.* **2013**, *7*, e2410. [CrossRef]

69. Richards, P.; Amara, J.; Ferme, M.C.; Mokuwa, E.; Sheriff, A.I.; Suluku, R.; Voors, M. Social pathways for Ebola virus disease in rural Sierra Leone, and some implications for containment. *PLoS Negl. Trop. Dis.* **2015**, *9*, e0003567. [CrossRef]

70. Sands, P.; Mundaca-Shah, C.; Dzau, V.J. The neglected dimension of global security—A framework for countering infectious-disease crises. *N. Eng. J. Med.* **2016**, *374*, 1281–1287. [CrossRef]

71. Global Health Security Agenda. 2024 Framework. Available online: https://www.ghsagenda.org/docs/default-source/default-document-library/ghsa-2024-files/ghsa-2024-framework.pdf?sfvrsn=4 (accessed on 30 March 2019).

72. Spengler, J.R.; Ervin, E.D.; Towner, J.S.; Rollin, P.E.; Nichol, S.T. Perspectives on West Africa Ebola virus disease outbreak, 2013–2016. *Emerg. Infect. Dis.* **2016**, *22*, 956–963. [CrossRef]

73. Pandey, A.; Atkins, K.E.; Medlock, J.; Wenzel, N.; Townsend, J.P.; Childs, J.E.; Nyenswah, T.G.; Ndeffo-Mbah, M.L.; Galvani, A.P. Strategies for containing Ebola in West Africa. *Science* **2014**, *346*, 991–995. [CrossRef]

74. World Health Organization. *Factors that Contributed to Undetected Spread of the Ebola Virus and Impeded Rapid Containment*; WHO: Geneva, Switzerland, 2015; Available online: https://www.who.int/csr/disease/ebola/one-year-report/factors/en/ (accessed on 17 March 2019).

75. DuBois, M.; Wake, C.; Sturridge, S.; Bennett, C. The Ebola response in West Africa: Exposing the Politics and Culture of International Aid. Available online: http://www.odi.org/publications/9936-ebola-response-west-africa-exposing-politics-culture-international-aid (accessed on 14 February 2019).

76. AlJezeera America. Saudi Arabia Announces 92 more MERS deaths, Sacks Deputy Health Minister. Available online: http://america.aljazeera.com/articles/2014/6/3/saudi-raises-mersdeathtollandcases.html (accessed on 17 March 2018).

77. The Guardian. China Accused of SARS Cover-up. Available online: http://www.theguardian.com/world/2003/apr/09/sars.china (accessed on 17 March 2019).

78. Convention on Biological Diversity. Nagoya Protocol. Available online: https://www.cbd.int/abs/about/ (accessed on 17 March 2019).

79. Institute of Medicine. *Enabling Rapid and Sustainable Public Health Research During Disasters: Summary of a Joint Workshop by the Institute of Medicine and the U.S. Department of Health and Human Services*; The National Academies Press: Washington, DC, USA, 2015; p. 190. [CrossRef]

80. Garrett, L. Ebola is back. And Trump is trying to kill funding for it. Available online: https://foreignpolicy.com/2018/05/09/ebola-is-back-and-trump-is-trying-to-kill-funding-for-it/ (accessed on 17 March 2019).

81. Kaiser Family Foundation. Trump administration requests rescission of $252M in 2015 Ebola funds as Congo addresses new outbreak. Available online: https://www.kff.org/news-summary/trump-administration-requests-rescission-of-252m-in-2015-ebola-funds-as-congo-addresses-new-outbreak/ (accessed on 17 March 2019).

82. Mills, J.N.; Ksiazek, T.G.; Peters, C.; Childs, J.E. Long-term studies of hantavirus reservoir populations in the southwestern United States: A synthesis. *Emerg. Infect. Dis.* **1999**, *5*, 135. [CrossRef]

83. Luis, A.D.; Kuenzi, A.J.; Mills, J.N. Species diversity concurrently dilutes and amplifies transmission in a zoonotic host–pathogen system through competing mechanisms. *Proc. Natl. Acad. Sci. USA* **2018**, *115*, 7979–7984. [CrossRef]

84. Luis, A.D.; Douglass, R.J.; Hudson, P.J.; Mills, J.N.; Bjørnstad, O.N. Sin nombre hantavirus decreases survival of male deer mice. *Oecologia* **2012**, *169*, 431–439. [CrossRef]

85. Bill and Melinda Gates Foundation. How We Work: Information Sharing Approach. Available online: https://www.gatesfoundation.org/How-We-Work/General-Information/Information-Sharing-Approach (accessed on 12 June 2018).

86. Bill and Melinda Gates Foundation. How we work: Open Access Policy. Available online: https://www.gatesfoundation.org/how-we-work/general-information/open-access-policy (accessed on 17 March 2019).

87. Wellcome Trust. Open Access Policy. Available online: https://wellcome.ac.uk/funding/managing-grant/open-access-policy (accessed on 2 February 2018).

88. Berger, K.M.; Schneck, P.A. National and transnational security implications of asymmetric access to and use of biological data. *Front. Bioeng. Biotechnol.* **2019**, *7*, 1–7. [CrossRef]

89. Wellcome Trust. Sharing Data During Zika and Other Global Health Emergencies. Available online: https://wellcome.ac.uk/news/sharing-data-during-zika-and-other-global-health-emergencies (accessed on 20 October 2018).

90. United Nations. About the Nagoya Protocol. Available online: https://www.cbd.int/abs/about/ (accessed on 14 August 2018).

91. World Health Organization. *Pandemic influenza preparedness Framework for sharing of influenza viruses and access to vaccines and other benefits*; WHO: Geneva, Switzerland, 2009. Available online: https://www.who.int/influenza/resources/pip_framework/en/ (accessed on 17 March 2019).

92. Ribeiro, C.D.; Koopmans, M.P.; Haringhuizen, G.B. Threats to timely sharing of pathogen sequence data. *Science* **2018**, *362*, 404–406. [CrossRef]

93. Christopher, M.M. One health, one literature: Weaving together veterinary and medical research. *Sci. Transl. Med.* **2015**, *7*, 303fs36. [CrossRef]

94. Hitziger, M.; Esposito, R.; Canali, M.; Aragrande, M.; Hasler, B.; Ruegg, S.R. Knowledge integration in one health policy formulation, implementation and evaluation. *Bull. World Health Organ.* **2018**, *96*, 211–218. [CrossRef]

95. Wellcome Trust. Sharing Research Findings and Data Relevant to the Ebola Outbreak in the Democratic Republic of Congo. Available online: https://wellcome.ac.uk/what-we-do/our-work/sharing-research-findings-and-data-relevant-ebola-outbreak-drc (accessed on 2 February 2018).

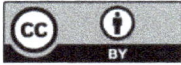

MDPI

St. Alban-Anlage 66

4052 Basel

Switzerland

Tel. +41 61 683 77 34

Fax +41 61 302 89 18

www.mdpi.com

Tropical Medicine and Infectious Disease Editorial Office

E-mail: tropicalmed@mdpi.com

www.mdpi.com/journal/tropicalmed

www.ingramcontent.com/pod-product-compliance
Lightning Source LLC
Chambersburg PA
CBHW051910210326
41597CB00033B/6090